Renal Diet

Cookbook

for Beginners

1500 days of easy-to-follow recipes with common ingredients low in sodium, potassium, and phosphorus to Protect Your Kidneys from More Damage. 28-Day Meal Plan Included

Kimberly Risner

HEALTHY
AIR FRYER RECIPES

TO DOWNLOAD THE FREE BONUS
SCAN THE QR CODE OR VISIT:

https://diamondpress.wixsite.com/kimberly-risner

Contents

INTRODUCTION

What is Renal Diet?

A renal diet is a diet low in sodium, phosphorus, and protein. People with kidney disease need to follow a renal diet because it can help slow the disease's progression. Kidney disease can lead to accumulation of toxins in the blood, and a renal diet can help to reduce this build-up. The diet may also help to reduce the amount of fluid retention in the body, which can lead to swelling. In addition, a renal diet can help to maintain healthy blood pressure levels. People with kidney disease often need to take medication to control their blood pressure, but following a renal diet can help to reduce the dosage of these medications.

If you suffer from kidney disease, you may wonder what changes your diet needs to be made. The positive news is that you can still enjoy many of your favorite foods, but there are a few things you should remember:

1. It is important to control your sodium intake. Excessive intake of sodium can cause fluid retention and high blood pressure, damaging the kidneys.
2. You need to limit your intake of phosphorus. Phosphorus is found in many foods but is especially abundant in dairy products, meat, and processed foods. Too much phosphorus can lead to calcium loss and weak bones.
3. You need to ensure you get enough vitamins and minerals.

Kidney disease can cause problems with absorption, so it is important to eat a balanced diet and take a multivitamin as directed by your doctor. Following these tips can help keep your kidneys healthy and prevent further damage.

How does Renal Diet work?

A renal diet is a diet that helps to support the health of the kidneys. The kidneys filter waste from the blood, so a renal diet works by focusing on foods that are low in sodium and potassium. This helps reduce the stress on the kidneys when they have to work, and can also help prevent or delay the onset of kidney disease.

Drinking plenty of fluids on a renal diet is important, as this helps flush out waste products from the body. Renal diets can be customized based on a person's needs, but some general guidelines are followed. If you are following a renal diet, it is important to speak with your doctor or registered dietitian to ensure that you get all the necessary nutrients you need.

How Nutrients are Regulated?

A renal diet is a special diet that helps protect your kidneys. The kidney is a very crucial organ in the body; its main job is to filter blood and remove the waste products from the body. When the kidneys are not working properly, wastes can lead to serious build-up in the blood and make you sick. A renal diet helps to prevent this by regulating the number of nutrients in the diet. The following are 10 ways nutrients are regulated in a renal diet:

Calories
Renal diets typically restrict calories to help manage weight and reduce stress on the kidneys.

Protein
Renal diets typically limit protein to help reduce waste products in the blood.

Fluid
Renal diets often restrict fluid to help prevent dehydration and reduce kidney stress.

Potassium

Renal diets typically restrict potassium to help prevent dangerous potassium levels in the blood.

Phosphorus

Renal diets typically restrict phosphorus to help prevent dangerous phosphorus levels in the blood.

Sodium

Renal diets typically restrict sodium to help prevent dangerous sodium levels in the blood.

Sugar

Renal diets often restrict sugar to help manage diabetes and reduce kidney stress.

Fat

Renal diets typically limit fat to help reduce waste products in the blood and improve heart health.

Alcohol

Renal diets typically recommend avoiding alcohol because it can harm the kidneys.

Caffeine

Renal diets typically recommend avoiding caffeine because it can harm the kidneys.

Benefits of Renal Diet:

A renal diet is a specific diet that helps kidneys function properly. The diet is intended for people with kidney disease, including eating restrictions and specific nutrient goals. Some of the benefits of following a renal diet are:

Reducing fluid retention

A key symptom of kidney disease is fluid retention, which can lead to swelling and high blood pressure. Following a renal diet helps to reduce fluid retention by limiting the intake of fluids and sodium.

Managing blood sugar levels

Kidney disease can cause blood sugar levels to rise, leading to diabetes. A renal diet helps to keep blood sugar levels in check by limiting sugar and carbohydrates.

Regulating blood pressure

High blood pressure is a common complication of kidney disease. A renal diet helps to lower blood pressure by reducing sodium and protein intake.

Preventing Anemia

Anemia is a specific type of common complication of kidney disease, and it can lead to fatigue and weakness. A renal diet helps to prevent anemia by ensuring adequate iron intake.

Preserving bone health

Kidney disease can cause bones to become weak and brittle. A renal diet helps to preserve bone health by ensuring adequate calcium and vitamin D intake.

Maintaining healthy cholesterol levels

Kidney disease can increase cholesterol levels, leading to heart disease. A renal diet helps to maintain healthy cholesterol levels by limiting saturated fat and cholesterol.

Promoting weight loss

Kidney disease often leads to weight gain, which can exacerbate other health problems. A renal diet promotes weight loss by limiting calories and unhealthy fats.

Preventing gastrointestinal problems

Kidney disease can cause gastrointestinal problems such as constipation and diarrhea. A renal diet helps to prevent these problems by ensuring adequate fiber intake.

Reducing inflammation

Inflammation is a common complication of kidney disease, and it can lead to pain and stiffness. A renal diet helps to reduce inflammation by limiting sodium and animal protein intake.

The benefits of a renal diet are numerous, making it an essential part of care for people with kidney disease.

Foods Allowed:

Renal diet is often recommended for people with kidney disease or kidney stones. While there are many restrictions on what you can eat on a renal diet, there are still plenty of delicious and nutritious foods to choose from. Here are some of the best:

Cauliflower

Cauliflower is a great source of fiber, vitamins, and minerals. It is low in potassium and phosphorus, making it an ideal food for people with kidney disease.

Broccoli

Like cauliflower, broccoli is a nutrient-rich vegetable low in potassium and phosphorus. It is also a good and healthy source of fiber and vitamin C.

Green beans

Green beans are a unique and nutritious vegetable that can be consumed cooked or raw. They are low in sodium and potassium and provide important vitamins and minerals.

Salmon

Salmon is an excellent and rich source of protein, omega-3 fatty acids, and vitamins D and B12. It is low in sodium and phosphorus, making it a great choice for people with kidney disease.

Chicken

Chicken is a lean source of low sodium and phosphorus protein. It can be enjoyed grilled, baked, or roasted for a healthy meal.

Quinoa

Quinoa is a nutritious grain high in protein and fiber. It is also low in sodium and potassium, making it a great option for people with kidney disease.

Greek yogurt

Greek yogurt provides calcium, protein, and probiotics for gut health. It is also low in sodium and potassium levels. Swap high-sodium yogurt products for Greek yogurt to get the same nutritional benefits without the risk of exacerbating kidney disease symptoms.

Egg whites

Egg whites are a good source of low sodium and phosphorus protein.

Canned tuna packed in water

Canned tuna is am convenient option when you want to get your seafood fix without having to cook anything. It's also low in sodium and contains no mercury, making it a safe choice for people with kidney disease.

Lean meats

Lean meats are yet another great source of protein for people with kidney disease. They are also low in toxins and other substances that can be hard on the kidneys.

Herbs

Herbs not only add flavor to food, but they also offer a variety of health benefits for people with kidney disease. They can help to improve circulation, boost immunity, and reduce inflammation throughout the body. Additionally, herbs are generally low in toxins and other substances that can be hard on the kidneys.

Water

Water is essential for everyone, but it is especially crucial for people with kidney disease since it helps to flush out waste products from the body. Drinking the required amount of water daily to stay hydrated and keep your kidneys healthy!

While there are many restrictions or what you can eat on a renal diet, these ten foods provide plenty of nutrients, taste and variety . Enjoy them as part of a healthy, balanced diet to help keep your kidneys functioning optimally.

Foods to Avoid

It is important to maintain a healthy diet if you have renal disease. This means avoiding foods that are high in salt, potassium, phosphorus, and fat. Here are some foods to avoid if you have a renal disease:

Processed meats

These meats are high in salt and phosphorus, which can aggravate kidney problems.

Canned soups

Most canned soups are also high in salt and phosphorus. Stick to low-sodium varieties or make your own soup at home.

Packaged snacks

Packaged snacks, such as chips and crackers, are loaded with salt and other unhealthy ingredients. Avoid these snacks altogether or choose healthier alternatives, such as nuts or seeds.

Frozen dinners

Most frozen dinners are also high in salt and phosphorus. Once again, it is best to stick to low-sodium varieties or make your own meals from scratch.

Cheese

Cheese is high in phosphorus, which can be dangerous for people with kidney problems. Choose low-fat cheeses or avoid cheese altogether.

Milk

Milk is also high in phosphorus, so it should be avoided or consumed in moderation by people with renal disease.

Dark chocolate

Chocolate is high in potassium, which can be considered dangerous for people with kidney problems. Choose milk chocolate instead or avoid chocolate altogether.

Dried fruits

Dried fruits are often very high in sugar, which can worsen kidney problems. Eat fresh fruit instead or choose sugar-free dried fruits.

Alcohol

Alcohol can worsen kidney problems and should be avoided by people with renal disease. If you still do drink alcohol, drink in moderation as well as stay hydrated.

Caffeinated beverages

Caffeinated beverages can also worsen kidney problems and should be avoided by people with renal disease. Stick to decaffeinated coffee and tea or water instead.

Precautionary Measures:

Anyone with kidney disease needs to be especially careful about what they eat and drink. That is because the kidneys might not be able to remove all the waste products from your blood. These waste products can build up and cause problems. Here are some precautionary measures for following a renal diet:

Limit your intake of protein

Protein is broken down into waste products that the kidneys have to filter, so it is important to limit your intake if you have kidney disease.

Eat plenty of fruits and vegetables

Fruits and vegetables are quite high in fiber, which helps to reduce the amount of waste that the kidneys have to filter.

Limit your intake of salt and sodium

Excessive salt can increase the amount of fluids in your body, which can put stress on the kidneys.

Drink plenty of fluids

Drinking fluids helps to flush waste products out of your body and prevent them from building up in your kidneys.

Avoid sugary drinks and foods

Sugar can increase the amount of waste in your blood, which can put strain on your kidneys.

Avoid alcohol

Alcohol can increase the risk of dehydration, which can strain your kidneys.

Exercise regularly

Exercise helps to keep your body healthy and reduces stress on your kidneys.

Quit smoking

Smoking cigarettes can damage your kidneys and make it harder for them to function properly.

Reduce your stress levels

If you are stressed out often or feel anxious frequently. Stress can worsen kidney function.

Get enough sleep every night

Lack of sleep can make it extremely difficult for your body to recover from illness or injury.

8 Diet tips to Help Prevent or Manage Chronic Kidney Disease:

Following these basic guidelines can help you maintain a healthy renal diet and protect your kidney function.

If you have chronic kidney disease, your diet plays an important role in managing the condition and preventing further damage to your kidneys. Here are eight diet tips to help you stay healthy:

1. Maintain a healthy weight.

Excess weight puts extra stress on your kidneys and can worsen chronic kidney disease. Talk to your doctor about a healthy weight for you, and aim to stay within that range.

2. Eat a balanced diet.

A diet that is rich in vegetables, fruits, and whole grains is good for your overall health and can also help protect your kidneys. Avoid all types of processed foods and foods high in saturated fat, salt, and sugar.

3. Limit your protein intake.

If you suffer from chronic kidney disease, your kidneys might be unable to process all the protein you eat. Consult your doctor about the amount of protein you consume eat each day, and choose a lean protein source like chicken or fish.

4. Limit your sodium intake.

Excessive can cause fluid retention and raise blood pressure, both of which can worsen chronic kidney disease. Avoid processed foods and fast food, and season your food on a daily basis with herbs and spices instead of salt.

5. Drink plenty of fluids.

Drinking enough fluids helps to flush waste products from your body and prevents dehydration. Discuss with your doctor about how much fluid you should be consuming each day, and make sure to drink even if you do not feel thirsty.

6. Get regular exercise.

Exercise can help control blood pressure and improve insulin resistance, which are risk factors for chronic kidney disease. Consult your doctor about what different types of exercise are safe for you, and aim for at least 30-40 minutes of moderate activity or exercise on most days of the week.

7. Quit smoking

Smoking is a major health hazard for chronic kidney disease, so quitting is essential for protecting your kidneys. Many resources are available to assist you in terms of leaving this habit; talk to your doctor about what would work best for you.

8. Monitoring your status with regular check-ups

Even if you are following all the diet tips above, monitoring your kidney function with regular check-ups is still important. This will help ensure that any early signs of kidney damage are detected so that treatment can be started as soon as possible.

FAQs

Renal diet is a type of diet that is typically recommended for people with kidney disease. The renal diet is aimed at helping to preserve normal kidney function and prevent further damage to the kidneys. There are a few key things you must know about the renal diet, which are discussed below.

What foods are restricted on a renal diet?

Foods that are high in phosphorus and potassium are typically restricted on a renal diet, as these minerals can be harmful to people with kidney disease. Examples of foods that are high in phosphorus and potassium include dairy products, meat, certain types of bears, and some vegetables

Why are phosphorus and potassium restricted on a renal diet?

Both phosphorus and potassium can be harmful to patients with kidney disease, as they can cause increased levels of calcium in the blood. High levels of calcium can lead to bone problems and other health complications.

What other dietary restrictions are there on a renal diet?

In addition to restricting phosphorus and potassium, a renal diet may also limit fluids, salt, and processed foods. This is because these can contribute to increased levels of stress on the kidneys.

What are the benefits of following a renal diet?

Following a renal diet can help maintain kidney function and prevent further kidney damage. Additionally, it can help to improve overall health by reducing the risk of complications like heart disease and stroke.

Who should follow a renal diet?

A renal diet is typically recommended for people with chronic kidney disease or Stage 4 or 5-kidney failure. However, it may also be recommended for people with other conditions that put stress on the kidneys, such as diabetes or hypertension. Consult your doctor if you believe you may benefit from following a renal diet.

BREAKFAST

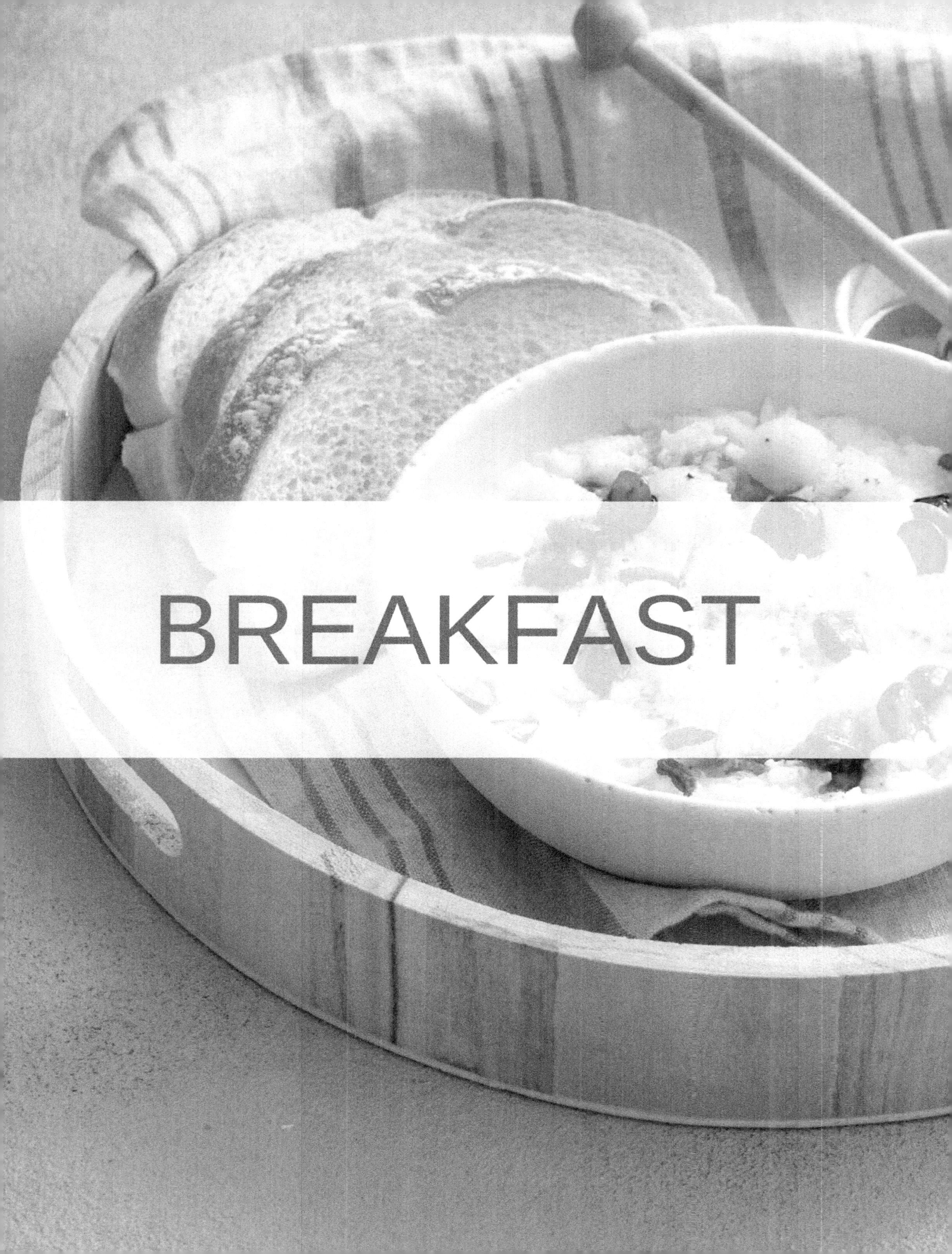

Raspberry Smoothie Bowl

Servings: 2 individuals
Preparation Time: 10 minutes

Ingredients:

- 2 cups frozen raspberries
- 1/3 cup fat-free milk
- ¼ cup fat-free plain Greek yogurt
- 2 tablespoons whey protein powder
- ¼ cup fresh raspberries

Instructions:

1. In a clean blender, add frozen raspberries and pulse for approximately 1 minute.
2. Add milk, yogurt and protein powder and pulse until desired consistency.
3. Transfer the mixture into 2 serving bowls evenly.
4. Serve with the topping of fresh raspberries.

Nutritional Information per Serving:

Calories: 118 - Fat: 1.2g - Sodium: 44mg - Carbohydrates: 20.2g - Fiber: 9g - Sugar: 9.4g - Protein: 8.5g

Fruity Yogurt Bowl

Servings: 4 individuals
Preparation Time: 10 minutes

Ingredients:

- 1 cup apples, peeled, cored and sliced
- 1 cup canned peaches, sliced
- 2½ cups fat-free plain Greek yogurt, divided
- 2 tablespoons maple syrup

Instructions:

1. In 4 serving bowls, divide the yogurt evenly.
2. Top with fruit slices and drizzle with maple syrup.
3. Serve immediately.

Nutritional Information per Serving:

Calories: 157 - Fat: 0.5g - Sodium: 64mg - Carbohydrates: 24.2g - Fiber: 1.9g - Sugar: 20.9g - Protein: 15.5g

Berries Cheese & Yogurt Bowl

Servings: 2 individuals
Preparation Time: 10 minutes

Ingredients:

- ½ cup fat-free plain Greek yogurt
- ½ cup low-fat cottage cheese
- 2 teaspoons olive oil
- ¼ teaspoon ground cinnamon
- ¼ cup fresh strawberries, hulled and sliced
- ¼ cup fresh blueberries
- ¼ cup fresh raspberries

Instructions:

1. In a large-sized bowl, add the yogurt, cheese, oil and cinnamon and mix until well blended.
2. Divide the yogurt mixture in 2 serving bowls.
3. Top with berries and serve immediately.

Nutritional Information per Serving:

Calories: 145 - Fat: 6.3g - Sodium: 194mg - Carbohydrates: 11.1g - Fiber: 2g - Sugar: 8.1g - Protein: 13g

Fruity Wheat Berries Bowl

Servings: 5 individuals
Preparation Time: 15 minutes
Cooking Time: 1 hour

Ingredients:

- 1½ cups water plus extra if needed
- ½ cup uncooked wheat berries
- 1 tablespoon canola oil
- 1 medium pear, cored and thinly sliced
- ½ cup fresh cranberries
- 1 teaspoon fresh ginger, finely grated
- 2 tablespoons maple syrup
- 1 teaspoon lemon zest, finely grated
- ½ teaspoon ground cinnamon

Instructions:

1. In a medium-sized, heavy-bottomed saucepan, add water and wheat berries over medium-high heat and bring it to a boil.
2. Now, reduce the heat to low and cook, covered for approximately 30 minutes.
3. Add extra water if needed and simmer for approximately 15-20 minutes or until desired doneness.
4. Meanwhile, in a wok, heat oil over medium heat.
5. Add pear slices and cook for approximately 3-4 minutes.
6. Add cranberries and ginger and cook for approximately 2-3 minutes.
7. Stir in cooked wheat berries, maple syrup, lemon zest and cinnamon and cook for approximately 1-2 minutes.
8. Serve warm.

Nutritional Information per Serving:

Calories: 91 - Fat: 3g - Sodium: 3mg - Carbohydrates: 15.7g - Fiber: 1.6g - Sugar: 7.9g - Protein: 1g

Cauliflower & Pear Porridge

Servings: 6 individuals
Preparation Time: 10 minutes
Cooking Time: 25 minutes

Ingredients:

- 2 cups pear, peeled, cored and shredded
- ½ cup low-fat unsweetened coconut, shredded
- ½ cup cauliflower rice
- 1¾ cups fat-free milk
- 1 teaspoon organic vanilla extract
- ¾ cup fresh strawberries, hulled and sliced

Instructions:

1. In a large-sized saucepan, stir together all ingredients except for strawberries over medium heat and bring it to a gentle boil.
2. Now, reduce the heat to low and simmer for approximately 15-20 minutes.
3. Serve warm with the topping of strawberries.

Nutritional Information per Serving:

Calories: 113 - Fat: 2.1g - Sodium: 64mg - Carbohydrates: 17.9g - Fiber: 2.9g - Sugar: 12.9g - Protein: 5.1g

Buckwheat Porridge

Servings: 2 individuals
Preparation Time: 10 minutes
Cooking Time: 15 minutes

Ingredients:

- 1 cup buckwheat, rinsed
- 1 cup fat-free milk
- 1 cup water
- ½ teaspoon ground cinnamon
- ½ teaspoon organic vanilla extract

- 1-2 tablespoons honey

Instructions:

1. In a saucepan, add all the ingredients except honey over medium-high heat and bring it to a boil.
1. Now, reduce the heat to low and cook, covered for approximately 10 minutes.
2. Stir in the honey and remove from heat.
3. Set aside, covered, for approximately 5 minutes.
4. With a fork, fluff the mixture and transfer into serving bowls.
5. Serve warm.

Nutritional Information per Serving:

Calories: 159 - Fat: 0.5g - Sodium: 72mg - Carbohydrates: 32g - Fiber: 2.6g - Sugar: 15.5g - Protein: 6.9g

Yogurt Oatmeal

Servings: 3 individuals
Preparation Time: 10 minutes
Cooking Time: 10 minutes

Ingredients:

- 2 cups water
- 1 cup gluten-free old-fashioned oats
- 7 ounces fat-free plain Greek yogurt
- 1¼ teaspoons ground cinnamon
- ¼ cup fresh blueberries

Instructions:

1. In a saucepan, add the water over medium heat and bring it to a boil.
2. Stir in the oats and cook for approximately 4-5 minutes, stirring occasionally.

3. Remove the pan of oats from heat and stir in half of the yogurt and cinnamon.
4. Divide the oatmeal into serving bowls evenly.
5. Top each bowl with the remaining yogurt and blueberries and serve

Nutritional Information per Serving:

Calories: 150 - Fat: 1.9g - Sodium: 40mg - Carbohydrates: 23.4g - Fiber: 3.5g - Sugar: 4.1g - Protein: 10.6g

Microwave Egg Whites Scramble

Servings: 2 individuals
Preparation Time: 10 minutes
Cooking Time: 1½ minutes

Ingredients:

- Olive oil cooking spray
- ¼ cup fat-free milk
- 6 egg whites
- ¼ cup fresh mushrooms, finely chopped
- Freshly ground black pepper, as required

Instructions:

1. Grease 2 (12-ounce) coffee mugs with cooking spray.
2. In a medium-sized glass bowl, add milk and egg whites and whisk until well blended.
3. Stir in mushrooms.
4. Divide the egg mixture into greased mugs evenly and microwave for approximately 45 seconds.
5. Remove the mugs from microwave and stir well.
6. Microwave for approximately 30-45 seconds more.
7. Serve immediately.

Nutritional Information per Serving:

Calories: 64 - Fat: 0.3g - Sodium: 94mg - Carbohydrates: 2.5g - Fiber: 0.1g - Sugar: 2.4g - Protein: 12.1g

Cheese & Egg Whites Scramble

Servings: 3 individuals
Preparation Time: 10 minutes
Cooking Time: 5 minutes

Ingredients:

- Olive oil cooking spray
- 8 egg whites, beaten
- 2 teaspoons dried dill weed
- Freshly ground black pepper, as required
- 3 tablespoons goat cheese, crumbled

Instructions:

1. Grease a non-stick wok with cooking spray and then heat over medium heat.
2. Add the beaten egg whites and sprinkle with dill weed and black pepper.
3. Cook for approximately 2-3 minutes, stirring continuously.
4. Remove from heat and immediately stir in cheese.
5. Serve immediately.

Nutritional Information per Serving:

Calories: 72 - Fat: 2.2g - Sodium: 124mg - Carbohydrates: 1.4g - Fiber: 0.1g - Sugar: 1g - Protein: 11.1g

Apple Omelet

Servings: 2 individuals
Preparation Time: 10 minutes
Cooking Time: 8 minutes

Ingredients:

- 6 egg whites
- ¼ cup fat-free milk
- 1 tablespoon water
- Freshly ground black pepper, as required
- 1 tablespoon olive oil
- 1 apple, peeled, cored and thinly sliced
- ¾ cup onion, thinly sliced
- 2 tablespoons part-skim mozzarella cheese, shredded

Instructions:

1. Preheat your oven to 400 °F.
2. In a glass bowl, add egg whites, milk, water and black pepper and whisk well.
3. In a small-sized ovenproof wok, heat oil over medium heat and sauté apple and onion for approximately 5-6 minutes.
4. With the spatula, spread the apple mixture in the bottom of wok.
5. Sprinkle with the cheese and top with egg mixture evenly.
6. Transfer the wok into the oven and bake for approximately 10-12 minutes.
7. Remove the wok from oven and cut the omelet into 2 equal-sized portions.
8. Serve warm.

Nutritional Information per Serving:

Calories: 218 - Fat: 8 7g - Sodium: 154mg - Carbohydrates: 21.7g - Fiber: 3.6g - Sugar: 15.6g - Protein: 14.6g

Zucchini Frittata

Servings: 6 individuals
Preparation Time: 10 minutes
Cooking Time: 20 minutes

Ingredients:

- 2 tablespoons fat-free milk
- 16 egg whites
- Freshly ground black pepper, as required
- 1 tablespoon olive oil
- 1 garlic clove, minced
- 2 medium zucchinis, cut into ¼-inch thick round slices
- ½ cup goat cheese, crumbled

Instructions:

1. Preheat your oven to 350 °F.
2. Add the milk, egg whites, and black pepper in a glass bowl and whisk well.
3. Heat the oil over medium heat in an ovenproof wok and sauté the garlic for approximately 1 minute.
4. Stir in the zucchini and cook for approximately 5 minutes.
5. Add the egg mixture and stir for approximately 1 minute.
6. Sprinkle the cheese on top evenly.
7. Immediately transfer the wok into the oven.
8. Bake for approximately 12 minutes or until eggs become set.
9. Remove the wok of frittata from oven and set aside to cool for approximately 5 minutes.
10. Cut into desired-sized wedges and serve.

Nutritional Information per Serving:

Calories: 112 - Fat: 5.3g - Sodium: 204mg - Carbohydrates: 3.8g - Fiber: 0.7g - Sugar: 2.5g - Protein: 12.4g

Apple Strata

Servings: 12 individuals
Preparation Time: 15 minutes
Cooking Time: 50 minutes

Ingredients:

- Olive oil cooking spray
- 1¼ cups fat-free milk
- 1¼ cups low-fat half-and-half creamer
- 1/3 cup unsalted margarine, melted
- ¼ cup pancake syrup
- 16 large egg whites
- 1 pound cinnamon bread loaf, cubed
- 8 ounces low-fat cream cheese, cubed
- 1 cup apple, peeled, cored and chopped
- 1 teaspoon ground cinnamon

Instructions:

1. Grease a large-sized baking dish with cooking spray.
2. In a bowl, add milk, half-and-half creamer, margarine, pancake syrup and egg whites and whisk until well blended. Set aside.
3. Place half of bread cubes evenly in the bottom of prepared baking dish, followed by cream cheese and apple.
4. Sprinkle with cinnamon and top with remaining bread cubes evenly.
5. Pour egg mixture on top evenly.
6. With plastic wrap, cover the baking dish and refrigerate overnight.
7. Preheat your oven to 325 °F.
8. Bake uncovered for approximately 50 minutes.
9. Remove from oven and set aside for approximately 5 minutes before serving.
10. Cut into 12 equal-sized wedges and serve.

Nutritional Information per Serving:

Calories: 264 - Fat: 10.5g - Sodium: 164mg - Carbohydrates: 30.8g - Fiber: 0.9g - Sugar: 5.4g - Protein: 11g

Cornmeal Waffles

Servings: 8 individuals
Preparation Time: 15 minutes
Cooking Time: 40 minutes

Ingredients:

- ½ cup warm water
- 2 envelopes active dry yeast
- 2 cups unsweetened rice milk
- ¼ cup olive oil
- 1 teaspoon white sugar
- 4 egg whites, lightly beaten
- 1½ cups all-purpose white flour
- ½ cup cornmeal
- Olive oil cooking spray

Instructions:

1. Add warm water and yeast in a large bowl and stir until dissolves completely.
2. Set aside for approximately 5 minutes.
3. Add rice milk, oil, and sugar and whisk until well blended.
4. Add egg whites, flour and cornmeal and whisk until just moistened.
5. Set the waffle mixture aside in a warm place for approximately 15 minutes.
6. Preheat the waffle iron and then grease it with cooking spray.
7. In preheated waffle iron, add the required amount of mixture and cook for approximately 4-5 minutes.
8. Repeat with the remaining mixture.
9. Serve warm.

Nutritional Information per Serving:

Calories: 193 - Fat: 7.4g - Sodium: 54mg - Carbohydrates: 27.5g - Fiber: 3g - Sugar: 0.7g - Protein: 5.7g

Chives Waffles

Servings: 10 individuals
Preparation Time: 15 minutes
Cooking Time: 50 minutes

Ingredients:

- 1½ cups all-purpose white flour
- 1 cup yellow cornmeal
- 2 tablespoons white sugar
- 2 teaspoons baking powder
- 1 teaspoon baking soda
- 2 teaspoons ground cumin
- ½ teaspoon red chili powder
- 1¾ cups fat-free milk
- 1/3 cup canola oil
- 4 egg whites
- 2 tablespoons fresh chives, minced
- Olive oil cooking spray

Instructions:

1. In a large-sized bowl, blend together flour, sugar, baking powder, baking soda and spices.
2. Add milk, oil, and egg whites in another bowl and whisk until well blended.
3. Add egg and milk into flour mixture and mix until well blended.
4. Fold in chives and set aside for approximately 10 minutes.
5. Preheat the waffle iron and then grease it with cooking spray.
6. In the preheated waffle iron, add about 1/3 cup mixture and cook for approximately 4-5 minutes.
7. Repeat with the remaining mixture.
8. Serve warm.

Nutritional Information per Serving:

Calories: 211 - Fat: 8g - Sodium: 144mg - Carbohydrates: 29g - Fiber: 1.5g - Sugar: 4.7g - Protein: 5.9g

Cottage Cheese Pancakes

Servings: 6 individuals
Preparation Time: 15 minutes
Cooking Time: 30 minutes

Ingredients:

- 1 cup low-fat cottage cheese
- ½ cup all-purpose white flour, sifted
- 1/3 cup unsalted butter, melted
- 8 egg whites, lightly beaten
- Olive oil cooking spray

Instructions:

1. In a bowl, add cheese, flour, butter and eggs and mix until well blended.
2. Lightly grease a non-stick wok with cooking spray and heat over medium-high heat.
3. Add about ¼ cup of mixture and the pan to spread in an even layer.
4. Cook for approximately 2-3 minutes.
5. Carefully flip the side and cook for approximately 1-2 minutes.
6. Repeat with the remaining mixture.
7. Serve warm.

Nutritional Information per Serving:

Calories: 185 - Fat: 11.1g - Sodium: 194mg - Carbohydrates: 9.7g - Fiber: 0.3g - Sugar: 0.5g - Protein: 11.2g

Vanilla Pancakes

Servings: 2 individuals
Preparation Time: 15 minutes
Cooking Time: 8 minutes

Ingredients:

- ¼ cup all-purpose white flour
- 1 teaspoon baking powder
- ¼ cup fat-free milk
- 6 egg whites
- 1 tablespoon maple syrup
- 1/8 teaspoon organic vanilla extract
- Olive oil cooking spray

Instructions:

1. In a large-sized bowl, blend together flour and baking powder.
2. Add remaining ingredients and mix until well blended.
3. Preheat the waffle iron and then grease it with cooking spray.
4. Place half of the mixture in the preheated waffle iron and cook for approximately 3-4 minutes or until golden brown.
5. Repeat with the remaining mixture.
6. Serve warm.

Nutritional Information per Serving:

Calories: 149 - Fat: 0.4g - Sodium: 114mg - Carbohydrates: 22.1g - Fiber: 0.5g - Sugar: 8.2g - Protein: 13.4g

Zucchini Muffins

Servings: 8 individuals
Preparation Time: 15 minutes
Cooking Time: 15 minutes

Ingredients:

- Olive oil cooking spray
- 8 egg whites
- ¼ cup unsalted butter, melted
- ¼ cup water
- 1/3 cup all-purpose white flour
- ½ teaspoon baking powder
- 1½ cups zucchini, grated
- ½ cup low-fat Parmesan cheese, shredded
- 1 tablespoon fresh oregano, minced
- 1 tablespoon fresh thyme, minced

Instructions:

1. Preheat your oven to 400 °F.
2. Lightly grease 8 cups of a muffin tin with cooking spray.
3. Add egg whites, butter and water in a large-sized bowl and whisk until well blended.
4. Add the flour and baking powder and blend well.
5. Add zucchini, Parmesan cheese and fresh herbs and mix until just combined.
6. Place the mixture into prepared muffin cups evenly and top with remaining cheese
7. Bake for approximately 13-15 minutes or until top of muffins become golden brown.
8. Remove the muffin tin from oven and place onto a wire rack to cool for approximately 10 minutes.
9. Then invert the muffins onto a platter and serve warm.

Nutritional Information per Serving:

Calories: 110 - Fat: 7.2g - Sodium: 134mg - Carbohydrates: 5.8g - Fiber: 0.8g - Sugar: 0.6g - Protein: 5.8g

Chicken Muffins

Servings: 8 individuals
Preparation Time: 10 minutes
Cooking Time: 20 minutes

Ingredients:

- Olive oil cooking pray
- 16 egg whites
- Freshly ground black pepper, as required
- 2 tablespoons water
- 8 ounces unsalted cooked chicken, finely chopped
- 1 cup bell pepper, seeded and chopped
- 1 cup onion, chopped

Instructions:

1. Preheat your oven to 350 °F.
2. Grease 8 cups of a muffin tin with cooking pray.
3. Add egg whites, black pepper, and water and whisk until well blended in a large-sized glass bowl.
4. Add chicken, bell pepper and onion and stir to blend.
5. Transfer the mixture in prepared muffin cups evenly.
6. Bake for approximately 18-20 minutes or until golden brown.
7. Remove the muffin tin from oven and place onto a wire rack to cool for approximately 10 minutes.
8. Then invert the muffins or to a platter and serve warm.

Nutritional Information per Serving:

Calories: 88 - Fat: 1g - Sodium: 65mg - Carbohydrates: 2.5g - Fiber: 0.5g - Sugar: 1.8g - Protein: 15.7g

Quinoa Bread

Servings: 12 individuals
Preparation Time: 15 minutes
Cooking Time: 1 hour

Ingredients:

- Olive oil cooking spray
- 2 cups uncooked quinoa rinsed
- 1 cup gluten-free oat flour
- 1 teaspoon baking soda
- 1 teaspoon baking powder
- ¼ teaspoon ground cinnamon
- 2 cups fat-free milk
- 3 tablespoons unsalted margarine melted
- 1 tablespoon fresh lemon juice

Instructions:

1. Preheat your oven to 400 °F.
2. Grease an 8x5-inch loaf pan with cooking spray.

3. In a food processor, add quinoa and pulse until a flour-like texture forms.
4. Transfer the quinoa flour into a large-sized bowl.
5. Add oat flour baking soda baking powder and cinnamon and mix well.
6. Add milk, margarine and lemon juice in another bowl and whisk until well blended.
7. Add the milk mixture into flour mixture and mix until well blended.
8. Place the mixture onto the prepared loaf pan evenly.
9. With a piece of foil, cover the loaf pan loosely.
10. Bake for approximately 30 minutes.
11. Now, remove the piece of foil and bake for approximately 30 minutes more.
12. Remove the loaf pan from oven and place onto a wire rack to cool for approximately 10 minutes.
13. Then invert the bread onto the wire rack to cool completely before slicing.

Instructions:

1. Preheat your oven to 350 ºF.
2. Line a loaf pan with baking paper.
3. In a food processor, add egg whites and pulse on high speed until frothy.
4. Add the remaining ingredients except for blueberries and pulse on high speed until smooth.
5. Transfer the mixture into a large-sized bowl and gently fold in the blueberries.
6. Place the mixture into the prepared loaf pan evenly.

14. Cut the bread into desired-sized slices and serve.

Nutritional Information per Serving:

Calories: 171 - Fat: 4.6g - Sodium: 134mg - Carbohydrates: 25.9g - Fiber: 2.9g - Sugar: 2g - Protein: 6.5g

Blueberry Bread

Servings: 8 individuals
Preparation Time: 15 minutes
Cooking Time: 45 minutes

Ingredients:

- 16 large egg whites, room temperature
- ¾ cup all-purpose white flour
- 1/3 cup unsalted butter, melted
- 1 teaspoon baking powder
- 1 teaspoon organic vanilla extract
- 1/3 cup fresh blueberries

7. Bake for approximately 40-45 minutes.
8. Remove the bread pan from oven and place onto a wire rack to cool for approximately 10 minutes.
9. Then invert the bread onto the wire rack to cool completely before slicing.
10. Cut the bread loaf into the desired-sized slices and serve.

Nutritional Information per Serving:

Calories: 150 - Fat: 7.9g - Sodium: 122mg - Carbohydrates: 10.7g - Fiber: 0.5g - Sugar: 1.2g - Protein: 8.5g

LUNCH

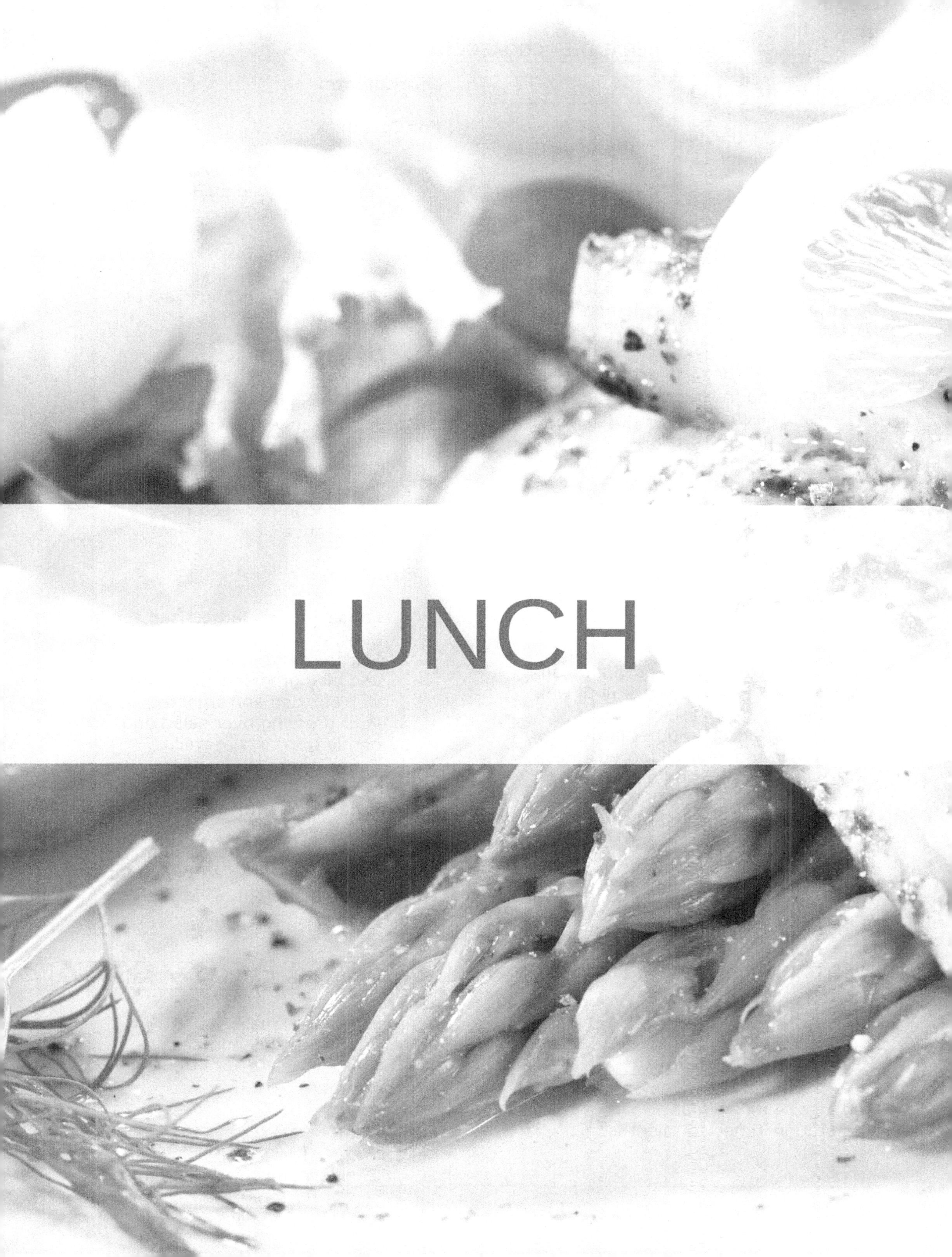

Mixed Fruit Salad

Servings: 12 individuals
Preparation Time: 15 minutes

Ingredients:

For Dressing:

- ½ cup fresh pineapple juice
- 2 tablespoons fresh lemon juice

For Salad:

- 1 pound fresh strawberries, hulled and sliced
- ½ pound fresh blackberries
- ½ pound fresh blueberries
- ½ pound seedless red grapes, halved
- ½ pound seedless green grapes, halved
- 4 fresh pears, cored and chopped
- 4 apples, pitted and chopped

Instructions:

1. For dressing: in a bowl, add all ingredients and whisk until well blended. Set aside.
2. For salad: in another large bowl, blend together all ingredients.
3. Add dressing and gently toss to coat well.
4. Refrigerate, covered to chill before serving.

Nutritional Information per Serving:

Calories: 142 - Fat: 0.5g - Sodium: 4mg - Carbohydrates: 35.5g - Fiber: 6.5g - Sugar: 25g - Protein: 1.4g

Papaya & Carrot Salad

Servings: 4 individuals
Preparation Time: 15 minutes

Ingredients:

For Salad:

- 2 large green papayas, peeled, seeded and julienned
- 2 large carrots, peeled and julienned
- 2 tablespoons fresh mint leaves, minced
- 2 tablespoons cilantro leaves, minced

For Dressing:

- ¼ cup shallot, finely chopped
- 2 garlic cloves, minced
- 1 Serrano pepper, seeded and chopped
- 2 tablespoons fresh lime juice
- 1 teaspoon unsweetened applesauce

Instructions:

1. For salad: in a large-sized serving bowl, add all ingredients and mix.
2. For dressing: in a food processor, add all ingredients and pulse until well blended and smooth.
3. Pour dressing over salad and gently toss to coat well.
4. Serve immediately.

Nutritional Information per Serving:

Calories: 95 - Fat: 0.5g - Sodium: 41mg - Carbohydrates: 23.4g - Fiber: 3.9g - Sugar: 14.3g - Protein: 1.5g

Watermelon & Cucumber Salad

Servings: 4 individuals
Preparation Time: 15 minutes

Ingredients:

For Vinaigrette:

- 2 tablespoons fresh lime juice

- 2 tablespoons honey
- 1 tablespoon olive oil

For Salad:

- 1 (5-pound) watermelon, peeled and cut into cubes
- 2 cups cucumber, cubed
- 3 tablespoons fresh mint leaves, torn
- ½ cup low-fat feta cheese, crumbled

Instructions:

1. For vinaigrette: in a small-sized bowl, all the ingredients and whisk until well blended.
2. In a large-sized bowl, add the watermelon, cucumber and mint and mix.
3. Place the vinaigrette and gently toss to coat.
4. Top with the feta cheese and serve.

Nutritional Information per Serving:

Calories: 182 - Fat: 4.2g - Sodium: 124mg - Carbohydrates: 35.7g - Fiber: 1.9g - Sugar: 29.5g - Protein: 4.6g

Broccoli & Cabbage Salad

Servings: 6 individuals
Preparation Time: 15 minutes

Ingredients:

For Dressing:

- 1 tablespoon shallot, minced
- 1/3 cup olive oil
- 2 tablespoons fresh lemon juice
- 1 teaspoon honey
- Freshly ground black pepper, as required

For Salad:

- 1½ cups broccoli florets, chopped
- 1½ cups cabbage, shredded
- 6 cups lettuce, chopped

Instructions:

1. For dressing: in a bowl, add all ingredients and whisk until well blended. Set aside.
2. For salad: in another large bowl, blend together all ingredients.
3. Add dressing and gently toss to coat well.
4. Serve immediately.

Nutritional Information per Serving:

Calories: 122 - Fat: 11.4g - Sodium: 15mg - Carbohydrates: 5.5g - Fiber: 1.4g - Sugar: 2.6g - Protein: 1.2g

Egg Drop Soup

Servings: 6 individuals
Preparation Time: 10 minutes
Cooking Time: 20 minutes

Ingredients:

- 1 tablespoon olive oil
- 1 tablespoon garlic, minced
- 6 cups salt-free chicken broth, divided
- 4 egg whites
- 1 tablespoon arrowroot powder
- 1/3 cup fresh lemon juice
- Freshly ground white pepper, as required
- ¼ cup scallion (green part), chopped

Instructions:

1. In a large-sized soup pan, heat the oil over medium-high heat and sauté garlic for approximately 1 minute.

2. Add 5½ cups of broth and bring it to a boil over high heat.
3. Adjust the heat to medium and cook for approximately 5 minutes.
4. Meanwhile, in a bowl, add egg whites, arrowroot powder, lemon juice, white pepper and remaining broth and whisk until well blended.
5. Slowly add egg mixture in the pan, stirring continuously.
6. Simmer for approximately 5-6 minutes or until desired thickness of soup, stirring continuously.
7. Serve hot with the garnishing of scallion.

Nutritional Information per Serving:

Calories: 79 - Fat: 17.5g - Sodium: 134mg - Carbohydrates: 2.6g - Fiber: 0.2g - Sugar: 0.6g - Protein: 7.7g

Asparagus Soup

Servings: 4 individuals
Preparation Time: 10 minutes
Cooking Time: 40 minutes

Ingredients:

- 1 tablespoon canola oil
- 3 scallions chopped
- 1½ pounds asparagus trimmed and chopped
- 4 cups salt-free vegetable broth
- Freshly ground black pepper, as required
- 2 tablespoons fresh lemon

Instructions:

1. In a large-sized saucepan, heat the canola oil over medium heat and cook the scallion for approximately 4-5 minutes.
2. Stir in the asparagus and broth and bring it to a boil.
3. Now, reduce the heat to low and cook, covered for 25-30 minutes.

4. Remove the soup pan from heat and set it aside to cool slightly.
5. Now, transfer the soup into a high-powered blender and pulse until finely smooth.
6. Return the soup into the same saucepan over medium heat and simmer for 4-5 minutes.
7. Stir in the lemon juice and black pepper and remove from heat.
8. Serve hot.

Nutritional Information per Serving:

Calories: 85 - Fat: 3.8g - Sodium: 37mg - Carbohydrates: 12.1g - Fiber: 3.9g - Sugar: 8.1g - Protein: 4.2g

Cauliflower Soup

Servings: 6 individuals
Preparation Time: 15 minutes
Cooking Time: 20 minutes

Ingredients:

- 2 cups cauliflower florets, chopped
- ½ cup carrot, peeled and chopped
- 1 cup onion, chopped
- 2 garlic cloves, minced
- 4½ cups salt-free vegetable broth
- Freshly ground black pepper, as required
- 2 ounces part-skim mozzarella cheese, shredded
- ¾ cup low-fat half-and-half creamer
- ¼ cup fresh parsley, chopped

Instructions:

1. In a large-sized soup pan, blend together cauliflower, carrot, onion, garlic, broth and black pepper.
2. Place the pan over medium-high heat and bring it to a boil.
3. Now, reduce the heat to low and simmer for approximately 10 minutes.

4. Remove the soup pan from heat and set it aside to cool slightly.
5. In a large-sized blender, add soup and pulse until smooth.
6. Return the soup into the pan over medium-low heat.
7. Stir in cheese and half-and-half and simmer for approximately 3-5 minutes or until heated completely.
8. Serve hot with the garnishing of parsley.

Nutritional Information per Serving:

Calories: 67 - Fat: 1.9g - Sodium: 94mg - Carbohydrates: 9.8g - Fiber: 1.6g - Sugar: 9.8g - Protein: 4.2g

Zucchini Noodles with Mushroom Sauce

Servings: 5 individuals
Preparation Time: 20 minutes
Cooking Time: 15 minutes

Ingredients:

- 1½ tablespoons olive oil
- 1 large garlic clove, minced
- 1¼ cups fresh button mushrooms, sliced
- ¼ cup salt-free vegetable broth
- ¼ cup low-fat sour cream
- Freshly ground black pepper, as required
- 3 large zucchinis, spiralized with blade C
- ¼ cup fresh parsley leaves, chopped

Instructions:

1. For mushroom sauce: in a large-sized wok, heat the oil over medium heat and sauté the garlic for approximately 1 minute.
2. Stir in the mushrooms and cook for approximately 6-8 minutes.

3. Stir in the broth and cook for approximately 2 minutes, stirring continuously.
4. Stir in the cream and black pepper and cook for approximately 1 minute.
5. Meanwhile, for the zucchini noodles: in a large-sized saucepan of boiling water, add the zucchini noodles and cook for approximately 2-3 minutes.
6. With a slotted spoon, transfer the zucchini noodles into a colander and immediately rinse thoroughly under cold running water.
7. Drain the zucchini noodles well and transfer onto a large-sized paper towel-lined plate to drain.
8. Divide the zucchini noodles onto serving plates evenly.
9. Remove the mushroom sauce from heat and place over zucchini noodles evenly.
10. Serve immediately with the garnishing of parsley.

Nutritional Information per Serving:

Calories: 88 - Fat: 5.4g - Sodium: 34mg - Carbohydrates: 8.9g - Fiber: 2.4g - Sugar: 4.7g - Protein: 3.4g

Stuffed Bell Peppers

Servings: 4 individuals
Preparation Time: 15 minutes
Cooking Time: 25 minutes

Ingredients:

- Olive oil cooking spray
- ½ pound fresh shitake mushrooms
- 1 cup celery stalk
- ½ cup onion, roughly chopped
- 2 garlic cloves, peeled
- 2 tablespoons olive oil
- Freshly ground black pepper, as required
- 4 small bell peppers, halved and seeded

Instructions:

1. Preheat your oven to 400 °F.
2. Grease a baking sheet with cooking spray.
3. Remove stem and seeds from each bell pepper.
4. In a food processor, add mushrooms, celery, onion, garlic, oil and black pepper and pulse until finely chopped.
5. Stuff the bell peppers with the mushroom mixture into the bell peppers.
6. Arrange the bell peppers onto the prepared baking sheet.
7. Bake for approximately 20-25 minutes or until slightly brown.
8. Serve warm.

Nutritional Information per Serving:

Calories: 141 - Fat: 7.5g - Sodium: 124mg - Carbohydrates: 19.4g - Fiber: 3.5g - Sugar: 9g - Protein: 2.5g

Stuffed Zucchini

Servings: 8 individuals
Preparation Time: 15 minutes
Cooking Time: 18 minutes

Ingredients:

- Olive oil cooking spray
- 4 medium zucchinis, halved lengthwise
- 1½ cups bell pepper, seeded and minced
- ½ cup fresh mushrooms, finely chopped
- 1 teaspoon garlic, minced
- 1 tablespoon dried oregano, crushed
- Freshly ground black pepper, as required
- ½ cup low-fat feta cheese, crumbled
- ¼ cup fresh parsley, finely chopped

Instructions:

1. Preheat your oven to 350 °F.
2. Grease a large-sized baking sheet with cooking spray.
3. With a small-sized spoon, scoop out the flesh of each zucchini half.
4. Discard the flesh.
5. In a bowl, blend together bell pepper, mushrooms, garlic, oregano and black pepper.
6. Stuff each zucchini half with the veggie mixture evenly.
7. Arrange zucchini halves onto the prepared baking sheet.
8. Bake for approximately 15 minutes.
9. Now, set the oven to broiler on high.
10. Top each zucchini half with feta cheese and broil for approximately 3 minutes.
11. Garnish with parsley and serve hot.

Nutritional Information per Serving:

Calories: 42 - Fat: 1.2g - Sodium: 94mg - Carbohydrates: 6g - Fiber: 2g - Sugar: 3g - Protein: 3.2g

Chicken & Pineapple Kabobs

Servings: 6 individuals
Preparation Time: 20 minutes
Cooking Time: 12 minutes

Ingredients:

- 2 tablespoons unsweetened applesauce
- 3 tablespoons balsamic vinegar
- 2 tablespoons olive oil
- 3 tablespoons fresh ginger, chopped
- 3 tablespoons fresh garlic, chopped
- 1 teaspoon red pepper flakes, crushed
- 3 cups skinless, boneless chicken, cubed
- 2½ cups fresh pineapple cubes

- 2 bell peppers, seeded and cubed

Instructions:

1. In a large-sized bowl, blend together the applesauce, vinegar, oil, ginger, garlic and red pepper flakes.
2. Add the chicken cubes and coat with marinade generously.
3. Refrigerate, covered for approximately 2-3 hours.
4. Preheat the grill to medium-high heat.
5. Grease the grill grate.
6. Thread chicken, pineapple and bell pepper onto metal skewers.
7. Place the chciken skewers onto the grill and cook for approximately 10-12 minutes or until desired doneness, flipping occasionally.
8. Serve hot.

Nutritional Information per Serving:

Calories: 195 - Fat: 7.6g - Sodium: 29mg - Carbohydrates: 16.1g - Fiber: 2.1g - Sugar: 9.5g - Protein: 17g

Shrimp & Watermelon Kabobs

Servings: 6 individuals
Preparation Time: 15 minutes
Cooking Time: 8 minutes

Ingredients:

- 1 jalapeño pepper, chopped
- 1 large garlic clove, chopped
- 1 (1-inch) piece fresh ginger, mined
- 1/3 cup fresh mint leave
- ½ cup water
- ¼ cup fresh lime juice
- 24 medium shrimp, peeled and deveined
- 4 cups seedless watermelon, cubed
- Olive oil cooking spray

Instructions:

1. In a food processor, add jalapeño, garlic, ginger, mint, water and lime juice and pulse until smooth.
2. Transfer the mint mixture into a large-sized bowl.
3. Add the shrimp and coat with marinade generously.
4. Cover the bowl of shrimp and refrigerate to marinate for at least 1-2 hours.
5. Preheat the grill to medium-high heat.
6. Grease the grill grate with cooking spray.
7. Remove shrimp from marinade and thread onto pre-soaked wooden skewers with watermelon.
8. Place the shrimp skewers onto the grill and cook for approximately 6-8 minutes or until done completely, flipping occasionally.
9. Serve hot.

Nutritional Information per Serving:

Calories: 163 - Fat: 2.1g - Sodium: 134mg - Carbohydrates: 3.5g - Fiber: 0.7g - Sugar: 4.8g - Protein: 26.5g

Chicken Pita Pizza

Servings: 2 individuals
Preparation Time: 15 minutes
Cooking Time: 13 minutes

Ingredients:

- Olive oil cooking spray
- 2 pita breads
- 3 tablespoons unsalted BBQ sauce
- 3 ounces unsalted cooked chicken, cubed
- ¼ cup onion, chopped
- 4 tablespoons low-fat feta cheese, crumbled

Instructions:

1. Preheat your oven to 350 °F.
2. Grease a baking sheet with cooking spray.
3. Arrange the pita breads onto the prepared baking sheet.
4. Spread the BBQ sauce over each pita bread evenly.
5. Top with chicken and onion evenly and sprinkle with cheese.
6. Bake for approximately 11-13 minutes.
7. Serve warm.

Nutritional Information per Serving:

Calories: 260 - Fat: 3.1g - Sodium: 114mg - Carbohydrates: 36g - Fiber: 2g - Sugar: 1.6g - Protein: 20g

Salmon Burgers

Servings: 5 individuals
Preparation Time: 15 minutes
Cooking Time: 7 minutes

Ingredients:

- 12 ounces unsalted cooked salmon, chopped
- ½ cup onion, minced
- 1 garlic clove, minced
- 3 egg whites
- ½ teaspoon paprika
- Freshly ground black pepper, as required
- 2 tablespoons olive oil
- 5 cups lettuce, torn

Instructions:

1. Preheat your oven to 350 °F.
2. Line a large-sized baking sheet with parchment paper.
3. In a large-sized mixing bowl, add all ingredients except for oil and lettuce and mix until well blended.
4. Make 10 equal-sized patties from mixture.

5. Arrange patties onto the prepared baking sheet in a single layer.
6. Bake for approximately 15 minutes.
7. Now, in a large-sized wok, heat oil over high heat.
8. Remove the salmon burgers from oven and transfer into the heated wok.
9. Cook for approximately 1 minute from both sides.
10. Divide lettuce onto serving plates evenly.
11. Place 2 burgers onto each plate and serve.

Nutritional Information per Serving:

Calories: 184 - Fat: 12.7g - Sodium: 39mg - Carbohydrates: 3.4g - Fiber: 0.7g - Sugar: 1.1g - Protein: 15.3g

Chicken Meatballs

Servings: 5 individuals
Preparation Time: 15 minutes
Cooking Time: 10 minutes

Ingredients:

- 1 pound ground chicken
- 2 garlic cloves, minced
- 2 large egg whites, beaten
- ½ cup low-fat Parmesan cheese, grated freshly
- 2 tablespoons fresh parsley, chopped
- Freshly ground black pepper, as required
- 2 tablespoons olive oil
- 5 cups lettuce, torn

Instructions:

1. In a large-sized bowl, add all ingredients except for butter and sesame seeds and with your hands, mix until well blended.

RENAL DIET COOKBOOK FOR BEGINNERS

2. Make small equal-sized balls from the mixture.
3. Heat olive oil in a non-stick sauté pan over medium heat and cook the meatballs for about 10 minutes or until done completely.
4. With a slotted spoon, transfer the meatballs onto a paper towel-lined plate to drain.
5. Divide lettuce onto serving plates evenly.
6. Top each plate with meatballs and serve.

Nutritional Information per Serving:

Calories: 236 - Fat: 14.2g - Sodium: 134mg - Carbohydrates: 2.4g - Fiber: 0.4g - Sugar: 0.7g - Protein: 23.1g

Beef & Veggie Meatballs

Servings: 5 individuals
Preparation Time: 15 minutes
Cooking Time: 30 minutes

Ingredients:

- ¾ cup carrot, peeled and grated
- ¾ cup zucchini, grated
- Pinch of salt
- 1 pound lean ground beef
- 1 egg, beaten
- ¼ of a small onion, finely chopped
- 1 garlic clove, minced
- 2 tablespoons fresh cilantro, finely chopped
- Freshly ground black pepper, as required
- 5 cups lettuce

Instructions:

1. Preheat your oven to 400 °F.
2. Line a large-sized baking sheet with parchment paper.
3. Arrange a large-sized colander in the sink. Add carrot and zucchini and sprinkle with 2 pinches of salt.

4. Set aside for at least 10 minutes.
5. Transfer the veggies over a paper towel and squeeze out all the moisture of veggies.
6. In a large-sized mixing bowl, add squeezed vegetables, beef, egg, onion, garlic, cilantro and black pepper and mix until well blenced.
7. Shape the mixture into equal-sized balls.
8. Place the beef meatballs onto the prepared baking sheet.
9. Bake for approximately 25-30 minutes or until done completely.
10. Divide lettuce onto serving plates evenly.
11. Top each plate with meatballs and serve.

Nutritional Information per Serving:

Calories: 162 - Fat: 7.5g - Sodium: 104mg - Carbohydrates: 4.5g - Fiber: 1.1g - Sugar: 1.9g - Protein: 19.6g

Asparagus Risotto

Servings: 4 individuals
Preparation Time: 15 minutes
Cooking Time: 45 minutes

Ingredients:

- 15-20 fresh asparagus spears, trimmed and cut into 1½-inch pieces
- 2 tablespoons olive oil
- 1 cup yellow onion, chopped
- 1 garlic clove, minced
- 1 cup Arborio rice, rinsed
- 1 tablespoon fresh lemon zest, grated finely
- 2 tablespoons fresh lemon juice
- 5½ cups hot salt-free chicken broth
- 1 tablespoon fresh parsley, chopped
- ¼ cup low-fat Parmesan cheese, grated

- Freshly ground black pepper, to taste

Instructions:

1. In a medium-sized saucepan of boiling water, cook the asparagus for approximately 3 minutes.
2. Drain the asparagus and rinse under cold running water.
3. Again, drain well and set aside.
4. In a large-sized saucepan, heat olive oil over medium heat and cook the onion for approximately 5 minutes.
5. Add the garlic and sauté for approximately 1 minute.
6. Add the rice and stir fry for approximately 2 minutes.
7. Add the lemon zest, lemon juice, and ½ cup of broth and cook for approximately 3 minutes or until all the liquid is absorbed, stirring gently.
8. Add 1 cup of broth and cook until all the broth is absorbed, stirring occasionally.
9. Repeat this process by adding ¾ cup of broth at a time until all the broth is absorbed, stirring occasionally. (This procedure will take about 20-30 minutes.)
10. Stir in the cooked asparagus and remaining ingredients and cook for approximately 4 minutes.
11. Serve hot.

Nutritional Information per Serving:

Calories: 314 - Fat: 28.1g - Sodium: 124mg - Carbohydrates: 44.9g - Fiber: 4g - Sugar: 3.2g - Protein: 12.6g

Buckwheat Noodles with Mushrooms

Servings: 4 individuals
Preparation Time: 15 minutes
Cooking Time: 8 minutes

Ingredients:

- 8 ounces buckwheat noodles
- 2 tablespoons olive oil
- 1 shallot, minced
- 3 cups fresh mushrooms, sliced
- ½ cup salt-free chicken broth

Instructions:

1. In a saucepan of boiling water, cook the noodles for approximately 5 minutes.
2. Drain the noodles well and rinse under cold water. Set aside.
3. Heat the oil in a large-sized wok over medium-high heat and sauté the shallot for approximately 3 minutes.
4. Add the mushrooms and stir fry for approximately 4-5 minutes.
5. Add the broth and simmer for approximately 2-3 minutes.
6. Add the noodles and cook for approximately 1-2 minutes, tossing occasionally.
7. Serve hot.

Nutritional Information per Serving:

Calories: 271 - Fat: 10g - Sodium: 41mg - Carbohydrates: 41g - Fiber: 3.6g - Sugar: 0.9g - Protein: 9.5g

Lemony Shrimp

Servings: 4 individuals
Preparation Time: 15 minutes
Cooking Time: 7 minutes

Ingredients:

- 2 tablespoons olive oil
- 1 pound medium shrimp, peeled and deveined
- 3 garlic cloves, minced
- Freshly ground black pepper, as required
- 1 tablespoon fresh lemon juice

Instructions:

1. Heat oil in a cast-iron wok over medium heat and cook the shrimp, garlic and black pepper for approximately 3 minutes per side, stirring occasionally.
2. Stir in the lemon juice and immediately remove from heat.
3. Serve hot.

Nutritional Information per Serving:

Calories: 172 - Fat: 8.4g - Sodium: 94mg - Carbohydrates: 0.8g - Fiber: 0.1g - Sugar: 0.1g - Protein: 24.5g

Scallops in Garlic Sauce

Servings: 5 individuals
Preparation Time: 15 minutes
Cooking Time: 13 minutes

Ingredients:

- 1¼ pounds fresh scallops, side muscles removed
- Freshly ground black pepper, as required
- 4 tablespoons unsalted butter, divided
- 5 garlic cloves, chopped
- ¼ cup salt-free chicken broth
- 1 cup low-fat sour cream
- 1 tablespoon fresh lemon juice
- 2 tablespoons fresh parsley, chopped

Instructions:

1. Sprinkle the scallops evenly with black pepper.
2. Melt 2 tablespoons of butter in a large-sized , non-stick wok over medium-high heat and cook the scallops for approximately 2-3 minutes per side.
3. Flip the scallops and cook for approximately 2 more minutes.
4. With a slotted spoon, transfer the scallops onto a plate.
5. Now, melt the remaining butter in the same wok over medium heat and sauté the garlic for approximately 1 minute.
6. Pour the broth and bring to a gentle boil.
7. Cook for approximately 2 minutes.
8. Stir in the cream and cook for approximately 1-2 minutes or until slightly thickened.
9. Stir in the cooked scallops and lemon juice and remove from heat.
10. Garnish with fresh parsley and serve hot.

Nutritional Information per Serving:

Calories: 237 - Fat: 14.1g - Sodium: 114mg - Carbohydrates: 8.7g - Fiber: 0.1g - Sugar: 3.3g - Protein: 21.2g

DINNER

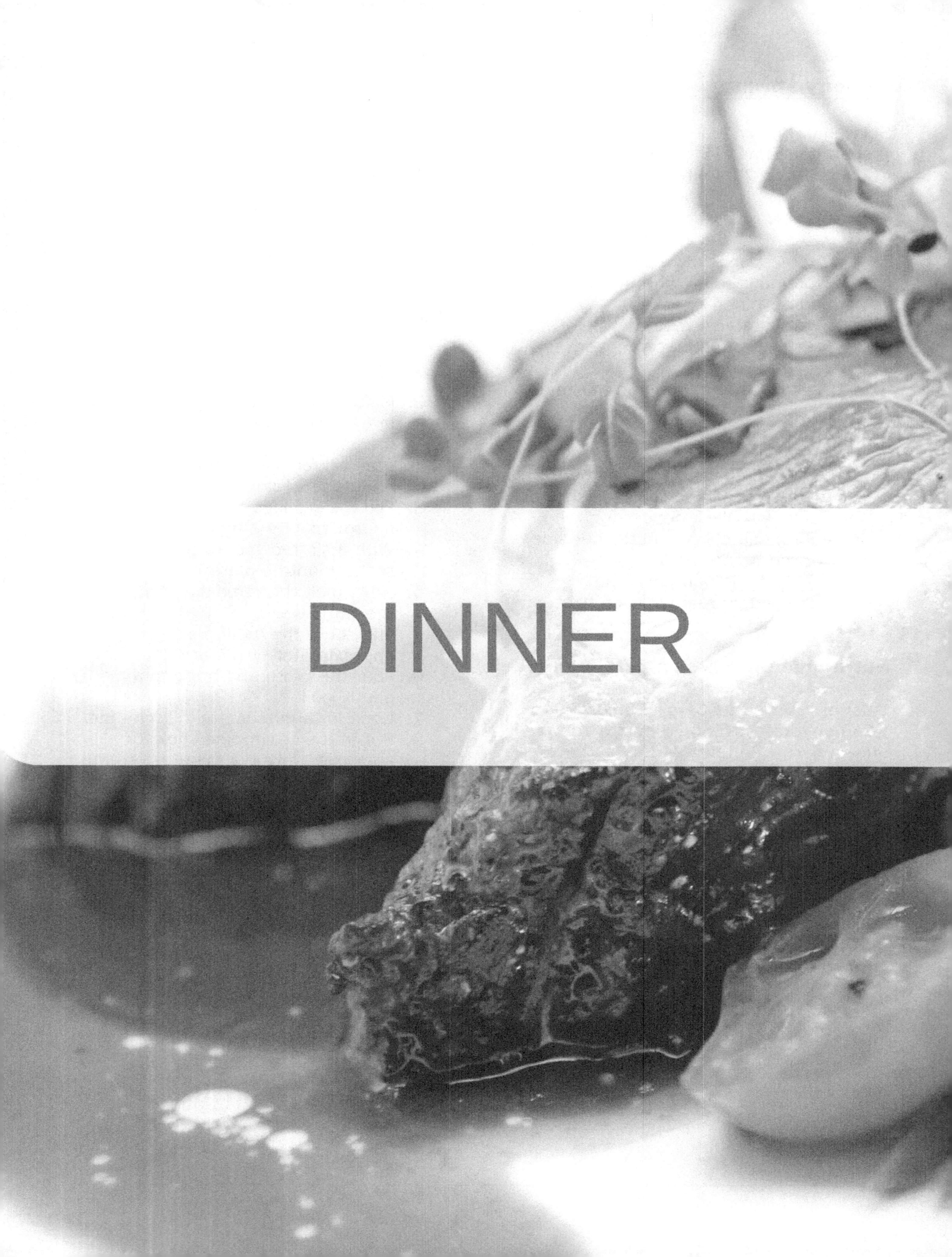

Chicken & Berries Salad

Servings: 6 individuals
Preparation Time: 15 minutes

Ingredients:

- 3 cups unsalted cooked chicken, chopped
- 1 cup fresh strawberries
- 1 cup fresh blueberries
- 1 cup fresh raspberries
- 6 cups lettuce, torn
- 2 tablespoons olive oil
- 2 tablespoons fresh lemon juice
- Freshly ground black pepper, as required

Instructions:

1. In a large-sized bowl, add all ingredients and gently stir to blend.
2. Serve immediately.

Nutritional Information per Serving:

Calories: 187 - Fat: 7.2g - Sodium: 49mg - Carbohydrates: 9.6g - Fiber: 2.8g - Sugar: 5.2g - Protein: 21.2g

Salmon & Cucumber Salad

Servings: 2 individuals
Preparation Time: 15 minutes

Ingredients:

- 6 ounces unsalted cooked salmon, chopped
- 1 cup cucumber, sliced
- 1 cup bell pepper, seeded and sliced
- 1 tablespoon scallion greens, chopped
- 2 cups lettuce, torn
- 1 tablespoon olive oil
- 1 tablespoon fresh lemon juice

Instructions:

1. In a salad bowl, place all ingredients and gently toss to coat well.
2. Serve immediately.

Nutritional Information per Serving:

Calories: 210 - Fat: 12.6g - Sodium: 45mg - Carbohydrates: 8.4g - Fiber: 1.5g - Sugar: 4.7g - Protein: 17.8g

Shrimp & Veggie Salad

Servings: 12 individuals
Preparation Time: 20 minutes

Ingredients:

For Dressing:

- 3 garlic cloves, minced
- ¼ cup fresh parsley, chopped
- 1 cup olive oil
- ½ cup fresh lemon juice
- ½ teaspoon dried oregano, crushed
- ½ teaspoon dried, crushed
- Freshly ground black pepper, as required

For Salad:

- 2 pounds unsalted cooked shrimp
- 4 cups cooked white rice
- 3 cups bell peppers, seeded and chopped
- 3 cups cucumber, chopped
- 1 cup onion, chopped
- 10 ounces pineapple, chopped
- ½ cup fresh cranberries
- ½ cup fresh parsley, minced
- 1/3 cup fresh dill weed, minced
- 16 cups lettuce, torn

Instructions:

1. In a bowl, add all dressing ingredients and whisk until well blended. Set aside.

2. In another large bowl, blend together all salad ingredients except lettuce.
3. Add dressing and gently toss to coat well.
4. Refrigerate, covered to chill completely.
5. Divide the lettuce into serving plates evenly.
6. Top with salad and serve.

Nutritional Information per Serving:

Calories: 344 - Fat: 1.68g - Sodium: 104mg - Carbohydrates: 25.4g - Fiber: 2.2g - Sugar: 5.8g - Protein: 20g

Chicken & Cabbage Soup

Servings: 4 individuals
Preparation Time: 15 minutes
Cooking Time: 25 minutes

Ingredients:

- 2 tablespoons olive oil
- ½ of medium onion, chopped
- 3 garlic cloves, minced
- 4½ cups salt-free chicken broth
- 2 cups cabbage, chopped finely
- 1 cup cooked chicken, cubed
- 2 tablespoons fresh lemon juice
- Freshly ground black pepper, to taste

Instructions:

1. In a soup pan, heat olive oil over medium-high heat and sauté the onion and garlic for approximately 4-5 minutes.
2. Stir in the cooked cabbage and broth and bring to a gentle boil.
3. Now, adjust the heat to low and cook for approximately 8-10 minutes.
4. Stir in the cooked chicken and simmer for 4-5 minutes.
5. Stir in the lemon juice and black pepper and remove from heat.
6. Serve hot.

Nutritional Information per Serving:

Calories: 172 - Fat: 25.1g - Sodium: 98mg - Carbohydrates: 4.2g - Fiber: 1.3g - Sugar: 1.9g - Protein: 16.6g

Ground Turkey & Cabbage Soup

Servings: 4 individuals
Preparation Time: 15 minutes
Cooking Time: 35 minutes

Ingredients:

- 2 teaspoons olive oil
- 12 ounces lean ground turkey
- ½ cup scallion, chopped
- 2 garlic cloves, minced
- 1 Serrano pepper, seeded and chopped
- 2 cups cabbage, shredded
- 4 cups salt-free chicken broth
- Freshly ground black pepper, as required

Instructions:

1. In a large-sized saucepan, heat olive oil over medium heat and cook the ground turkey for approximately 6-7 minutes.
2. Add scallion and garlic and sauté for approximately 2-3 minutes.
3. Drain off excess fat from pan.
4. Add cabbage and broth and bring it to a boil.
5. Now, reduce the heat to low and cook, covered for approximately 15-20 minutes or until desired doneness.
6. Stir in black pepper and remove from heat.
7. Serve hot.

Nutritional Information per Serving:

Calories: 192 - Fat: 23.5g - Sodium: 99mg - Carbohydrates: 3.6g - Fiber: 1.3g - Sugar: 1.5g - Protein: 22.5g

Salmon Soup

Servings: 4 individuals
Preparation Time: 15 minutes
Cooking Time: 30 minutes

Ingredients:

- 2 tablespoons olive oil
- 2 garlic cloves, minced
- 1 head cabbage, chopped
- 4 cups salt-free chicken broth
- ¼ cup fresh cilantro, minced
- Freshly ground black pepper, as required
- 1 shallot, chopped
- 1 jalapeño pepper, chopped
- 2 small bell peppers, seeded and chopped
- 3 (4-ounce) boneless salmon fillets, cubed
- 2 tablespoons fresh lemon juice

Instructions:

1. Heat olive oil in a large-sized soup pan over medium heat and sauté shallot and garlic for approximately 2-3 minutes.
2. Add cabbage and bell peppers and sauté for approximately 3-4 minutes.
3. Add broth and bring it to a boil over high heat.
4. Now, reduce the heat to medium-low and simmer for approximately 10 minutes.
5. Add salmon and cook for approximately 5-6 minutes.
6. Stir in the cilantro, lemon juice and black pepper and cook for approximately 2 minutes.
7. Serve hot.

Nutritional Information per Serving:

Calories: 260 - Fat: 12.7g - Sodium: 94mg - Carbohydrates: 21g - Fiber: 5.5g - Sugar: 13.4g - Protein: 19.9g

Chicken & Cauliflower Stew

Servings: 6 individuals
Preparation Time: 15 minutes
Cooking Time: 40 minutes

Ingredients:

- 2 tablespoons olive oil
- 1 onion, chopped
- 1 carrot, peeled and chopped
- 1 tablespoon garlic, minced
- 1 tablespoon fresh ginger, minced
- 1 teaspoon ground turmeric
- 1 teaspoon ground cumin
- 1 teaspoon ground coriander
- 1 teaspoon paprika
- 4 (5-ounce) boneless, skinless chicken thighs, cut into 1-inch pieces
- 4 cups cauliflower, cut into small florets
- 3 cups salt-free chicken broth
- Freshly ground black pepper, as required
- 2 tablespoons fresh lemon juice

Instructions:

1. Heat oil in a large-sized heavy-bottomed pan over medium heat and sauté the onion for approximately 3-4 minutes.
2. Add the ginger, garlic, and spices, and sauté for approximately 1 minute.
3. Add the chicken and cook for approximately 4-5 minutes.
4. Add the cauliflower, broth and black pepper and bring it to a gentle simmer.
5. Now, adjust the heat to low and cook, covered for approximately 20-25 minutes.
6. Add in lemon juice and remove from heat.
7. Serve hot.

Nutritional Information per Serving:

Calories: 275 - Fat: 19.5g - Sodium:

100mg - Carbohydrates: 8.1g - Fiber: 2.7g - Sugar: 3.1g - Protein: 31.8g

Baked Beef Stew

Servings: 8 individuals
Preparation Time: 15 minutes
Cooking Time: 25 minutes

Ingredients:

- 1 cup water
- 3 tablespoons arrowroot starch
- 1 (1½-pound) beef chuck roast, trimmed and cubed
- 1 pound fresh mushrooms, sliced
- 4 medium carrots, peeled and chopped
- 3 celery stalks, chopped
- 2 medium onions, chopped
- 1 tablespoon fresh thyme, chopped
- 2 garlic cloves, minced
- 2 cups salt-free chicken broth
- Freshly ground black pepper, as required

Instructions:

1. Preheat your oven to 325 °F.
2. In a bowl, blend together water and arrowroot starch.
3. In a large-sized oven-proof pan, add remaining ingredients and stir to blend.
4. Slowly add arrowroot starch mixture, stirring continuously.
5. Cover the pan and bake for approximately 3 hours, stirring after every 30 minutes.
6. Serve hot.

Nutritional Information per Serving:

Calories: 221 - Fat: 12.4g - Sodium: 84mg - Carbohydrates: 10.7g - Fiber: 2.3g - Sugar: 3.8g - Protein: 27.6g

Salmon & Shrimp Stew

Servings: 10 individuals
Preparation Time: 15 minutes
Cooking Time: 25 minutes

Ingredients:

- 2 tablespoons olive oil
- 2 cups onion, finely chopped
- 2 garlic cloves, minced
- 1 Serrano pepper, chopped
- 1 teaspoon smoked paprika
- 4-5 cups salt-free chicken broth
- 1 pound salmon fillets, cubed
- 1 pound shrimp, peeled and deveined
- 2 tablespoons fresh lime juice
- Freshly ground black pepper, as required
- ¼ cup fresh parsley, chopped

Instructions:

1. In a large-sized soup pan, heat oil over medium-high heat and sauté the onion for approximately 5 minutes.
2. Add the garlic, Serrano pepper, and paprika, and sauté for approximately 1 minute.
3. Add in broth and bring it to a boil.
4. Adjust the heat to medium and simmer for approximately 5 minutes.
5. Add the salmon and simmer for approximately 3-4 minutes.
6. Stir in the shrimp and cook for approximately 4-5 minutes.
7. Stir in lemon juice and black pepper, and serve hot with the garnishing of parsley.

Nutritional Information per Serving:

Calories: 164 - Fat: 12.4g - Sodium: 102mg - Carbohydrates: 3.3g - Fiber: 0.7g - Sugar: 1g - Protein: 21.5g

Turkey & Zucchini Chili

Servings: 10 individuals
Preparation Time: 15 minutes
Cooking Time: 2 hours 20 minutes

Ingredients:

- 2 tablespoons olive oil
- 1 large onion, chopped
- 1 large bell pepper, seeded and chopped
- 4 garlic cloves, minced
- 1 jalapeño pepper, chopped
- 1 teaspoon dried basil, crushed
- 1 teaspoon dried thyme, crushed
- 1 tablespoon red chili powder
- 1 tablespoon ground cumin
- 2 pounds lean ground turkey
- 2 cup zucchini, chopped
- 2 cups salt-free chicken broth
- 2 cups water
- 1 cup scallion, chopped

Instructions:

1. In a large-sized saucepan, heat oil over medium heat and cook onion and bell pepper for approximately 5-7 minutes.
2. Add garlic, jalapeño pepper, herbs, spices and black pepper and sauté for approximately 1 minute.
3. Add turkey and cook for approximately 4-5 minutes.
4. Stir in zucchini and cook for approximately 2 minutes.
5. Add broth and water and bring it to a boil.
6. Now, reduce the heat to low and cook, covered for approximately 2 hours.
7. Serve hot with the garnishing of scallion.

Nutritional Information per Serving:

Calories: 184 - Fat: 12.7g - Sodium: 92mg - Carbohydrates: 5g - Fiber: 1.4g - Sugar: 2g - Protein: 19.9g

Chicken in Dill Sauce

Servings: 6 individuals
Preparation Time: 15 minutes
Cooking Time: 1 hour 5 minutes

Ingredients:

- 6 skinless, bone-in chicken thighs
- Freshly ground black pepper, as required
- 2 tablespoons olive oil
- ½ of medium onion, sliced
- 4 cups salt-free chicken broth
- 8 fresh dill sprigs
- ½ teaspoon cayenne powder
- ½ teaspoon ground turmeric
- 2 tablespoons fresh lemon juice
- 2 tablespoons cornstarch
- 1 tablespoon cold water
- 3 tablespoons fresh dill, chopped

Instructions:

1. Season the chicken thighs with black pepper.
2. In a large-sized Dutch oven, heat the oil over high heat.
3. In the pan, place chicken thighs, skin-side down and cook for approximately 4 minutes.
4. Transfer the chicken thighs onto a plate.
5. In the same Dutch oven, add the onion over medium heat and sauté for approximately 5-7 minutes.
6. Now, place the chicken thighs, skin side up, and sprinkle with cayenne powder and turmeric.
7. Top with broth and dill sprigs and bring it to a boil.
8. Now, reduce the heat to medium-low and cook, covered, for approximately 40-45 minutes, coating the thighs with cooking liquid occasionally.
9. Discard the thyme sprigs and transfer the thighs into a bowl.
10. Add the lemon juice, salt, and black pepper and stir to blend.

11. In a small-sized bowl, dissolve the cornstarch into water.
12. Slowly add the cornstarch mixture into the pan, stirring continuously.
13. Cook for approximately 3-4 minutes, stirring frequently.
14. Pour sauce over thighs and serve hot with a sprinkling of chopped dill.

Nutritional Information per Serving:

Calories: 279 - Fat: 21.6g - Sodium: 124mg - Carbohydrates: 4.5g - Fiber: 0.5g - Sugar: 0.5g - Protein: 36.9g

Chicken with Veggies

Servings: 6 individuals
Preparation Time: 15 minutes
Cooking Time: 15 minutes

Ingredients:

- 4 teaspoons olive oil, divided
- 1 pound skinless, boneless chicken tenders, cubed
- 1 teaspoon fresh ginger, minced
- 2 garlic cloves, minced
- ¾ teaspoon red pepper flakes, crushed
- 1/3 cup water, divided
- 1½ teaspoons cornstarch
- 3 cups broccoli, cut into bite-sized pieces
- 3 cup bell pepper, seeded and sliced

Instructions:

1. In a large-sized non-stick wok, heat 2 teaspoons of olive oil over high heat and cook chicken for approximately 6-8 minutes, stirring frequently.
2. Transfer the chicken into a bowl.
3. In the same wok, heat remaining olive oil over medium heat and sauté ginger, garlic and red pepper flakes for approximately 1 minute.

4. Add ¼ cup of water, broccoli and bell pepper and stir fry for approximately 2-3 minutes.
5. Meanwhile, in a small-sized bowl, dissolve the cornstarch in the remaining water.
6. Stir in chicken and cornstarch mixture and cook for approximately 2-3 minutes.
7. Serve hot.

Nutritional Information per Serving:

Calories: 161 - Fat: 6.2g - Sodium: 44mg - Carbohydrates: 8.8g - Fiber: 2.1g - Sugar: 3.8g - Protein: 18.9g

Ground Turkey with Veggies

Servings: 6 individuals
Preparation Time: 15 minutes
Cooking Time: 25 minutes

Ingredients:

- 1¼ pounds lean ground turkey
- 2 tablespoons olive oil
- 1 medium onion, chopped
- 2 cups carrot, peeled and chopped
- 6 garlic cloves, minced
- 2 cups asparagus, trimmed and cut into 1-inch pieces
- ¼ cup salt-free chicken broth
- ¼ teaspoon red pepper flakes, crushed
- Freshly ground black pepper, as required

Instructions:

1. Heat a non-stick wok over medium-high heat and cook the turkey for approximately 6-8 minutes or until browned.
2. With a slotted spoon, transfer the turkey in a bowl and discard the grease from wok.
3. In the same wok, heat olive oil over medium heat and sauté

onion, carrot and garlic for approximately 5 minutes

4. Add asparagus and cooked turkey and stir to blend.
5. Add the broth, red pepper flakes and black pepper and bring it to a boil.
6. Now adjust the heat to medium-low and cook for approximately 6-8 minutes, stirring frequently.
7. Serve hot.

Nutritional Information per Serving:

Calories: 213 - Fat: 12.2g - Sodium: 94mg - Carbohydrates: 8.1g - Fiber: 2.3g - Sugar: 3.5g - Protein: 20.5g

Beef Casserole

Servings: 12 individuals
Preparation Time: 15 minutes
Cooking Time: 57 minutes

Ingredients:

- Olive oil cooking spray
- 2 pounds lean ground beef
- ½ cup onion, chopped
- ½ teaspoon garlic, minced
- Freshly ground black pepper, as required
- 8 ounces part-skim mozzarella cheese, shredded and divided
- 2 egg whites, beaten
- 16 ounces frozen green beans
- 3 tablespoons unsalted butter, divided
- 16 ounces frozen cauliflower
- ¼ cup low-fat sour cream

Instructions:

1. Preheat your oven to 350 °F.
2. Lightly grease a large-sized baking dish with cooking spray.
3. Heat a large-sized non-stick wok over medium-high heat and cook the beef for approximately 4-5 minutes.

4. Add onion and garlic and cook for approximately 4-5 minutes. Drain the excess grease from pan.
5. Stir in black pepper and remove from heat.
6. Stir in ½ of cheese and egg whites and transfer into a baking dish.
7. Meanwhile, add green beans in a saucepan of boiling water and cook for approximately 4-5 minutes.
8. Drain the green beans well and transfer into a bowl.
9. Add 1 tablespoon of butter and stir to blend.
10. In the same pan, add cauliflower and boil for approximately 10-12 minutes.
11. Drain well.
12. Add cauliflower, sour cream, remaining butter, and black pepper in a clean food processor and pulse until smooth.
13. Place green beans over beef mixture evenly and top with cauliflower mixture.
14. Sprinkle with the remaining cheese evenly.
15. Bake for approximately 35 minutes or until bubbly.
16. Remove the baking dish from oven and set aside for approximately 10 minutes before serving.

Nutritional Information per Serving:

Calories: 223 - Fat: 12.7g - Sodium: 104mg - Carbohydrates: 6.1g - Fiber: 2.3g - Sugar: 1.7g - Protein: 22.5g

Ground Beef with Mushrooms

Servings: 4 individuals
Preparation Time: 15 minutes
Cooking Time: 28 minutes

Ingredients:

- ¾ pound lean ground beef
- 2 tablespoons olive oil

- 2 garlic cloves, minced
- ½ of onion, chopped
- 2 cups fresh mushrooms, sliced
- 2 tablespoons fresh basil
- ¼ cup salt-free chicken broth
- 2 tablespoons balsamic vinegar
- 2 tablespoons fresh parsley, chopped

Instructions:

1. Heat a large-sized non-stick wok over medium-high heat and cook the ground beef for approximately 8-10 minutes, breaking up the chunks with a wooden spoon.
2. With a slotted spoon, transfer the beef into a bowl.
3. In the same wok, add the onion and garlic for approximately 3 minutes.
4. Add the mushrooms and cook for approximately 5-7 minutes
5. Add the cooked beef, basil, broth and vinegar and bring it to a boil
6. Adjust the heat to medium-low and simmer for approximately 3 minutes.
7. Stir in parsley and serve immediately.

Nutritional Information per Serving:

Calories: 202 - Fat: 14.2g - Sodium: 77mg - Carbohydrates: 3.2g - Fiber: 0.8g - Sugar: 1.3g - Protein: 18.5g

Salmon in Yogurt Sauce

Servings: 6 individuals
Preparation Time: 15 minutes
Cooking Time: 30 minutes

Ingredients:

- 6 (4-ounce) skinless salmon fillets
- 1½ teaspoons ground turmeric, divided
- 3 tablespoons canola oil, divided
- 1 (1-inch) stick cinnamon, pounded roughly

- 3-4 green cardamom, pounded roughly
- 2 bay leaves
- 1 onion, chopped finely
- 1 teaspoon garlic paste
- 1½ teaspoons ginger paste
- 3-4 green chilies, halved
- ¾ cup fat-free plain Greek yogurt
- ¾ cup water
- 3 tablespoons fresh cilantro, chopped

Instructions:

1. Rub the salmon with ½ teaspoon of turmeric and set aside.
2. Heat 1½-2 tablespoons of canola oil in a large-sized, non-stick wok over medium heat and cook salmon fillets for approximately 2 minutes per side.
3. Transfer the salmon steaks into a bowl.
4. In the same wok, melt the remaining oil over medium heat and sauté cinnamon, green cardamom, whole cloves and bay leaves for approximately 1 minute.
5. Add onion and sauté for approximately 4-5 minutes.
6. Add garlic paste, ginger paste, green chilies and turmeric and sauté for approximately 2 minutes.
7. Meanwhile, in a bowl, add yogurt and water and whisk until smooth.
8. Now adjust the heat to low and slowly, add the yogurt mixture, stirring continuously.
9. Simmer, covered for approximately 15 minutes.
10. Carefully add the salmon fillets and simmer for approximately 5 minutes.
11. Serve hot with the topping of cilantro.

Nutritional Information per Serving:

Calories: 295 - Fat: 19.3g - Sodium: 82mg - Carbohydrates: 4.8g - Fiber: 0.9g - Sugar: 2g - Protein: 25.6g

Cod & Mushroom Casserole

Servings: 4 individuals
Preparation Time: 15 minutes
Cooking Time: 21 minutes

Ingredients:

- 2 tablespoons unsalted margarine
- ¼ cup onion, chopped
- 1½ cups fresh mushrooms, sliced
- 1 pound fresh cod fillets
- Freshly ground black pepper, as required
- 1 teaspoon dried thyme, crushed

Instructions:

1. Preheat your oven to 450 °F.
2. In a wok, melt margarine over medium heat.
3. Add onion and mushrooms and sauté for approximately 5-6 minutes.
4. Arrange the cod fillets into a large-sized baking dish and top with the mushroom mixture evenly.
5. Sprinkle with black pepper and thyme
6. Bake for approximately 12-15 minutes.
7. Serve hot.

Nutritional Information per Serving:

Calories: 150 - Fat: 6.8g - Sodium: 94mg - Carbohydrates: 1.6g - Fiber: 0.4g - Sugar: 0.8g - Protein: 21.2g

Shrimp with Veggies

Servings: 6 individuals
Preparation Time: 20 minutes
Cooking Time: 10 minutes

Ingredients:

- 2 tablespoons olive oil, divided

- 1 pound large shrimp, peeled and deveined
- ½ of onion, chopped
- 3 garlic cloves, minced
- 2 cups broccoli floret
- 2 cups carrot, peeled and julienned
- 2-3 tablespoons salt-free chicken broth
- Freshly ground black pepper, as required
- 2 tablespoons fresh parsley, chopped

Instructions:

1. In a large-sized non-stick wok, heat 1 tablespoon of olive oil over medium heat and stir fry the shrimp for approximately 1 minute per side.
2. With a slotted spoon, transfer the shrimp onto a plate.
3. In the same wok, heat remaining olive oil over medium heat and sauté the onion and garlic for approximately 2-3 minutes.
4. Add the vegetables, broth and black pepper and stir fry for approximately 2-3 minutes.
5. Stir in the cooked shrimp and stir fry for approximately 1-2 minutes.
6. Serve hot.

Nutritional Information per Serving:

Calories: 133 - Fat: 5.1g - Sodium: 84mg - Carbohydrates: 8.4g - Fiber: 2g - Sugar: 2.7g - Protein: 15.7g

Curried Veggies Bake

Servings: 6 individuals
Preparation Time: 15 minutes
Cooking Time: 20 minutes

Ingredients:

- 1 eggplant, cubed
- 1 small zucchini, chopped
- 1 small yellow squash, chopped

- 2 bell peppers, seeded and cubed
- 1 onion, thinly sliced
- 1 tablespoon maple syrup
- 2 tablespoons canola oil
- 2 teaspoons salt-free curry powder
- Freshly ground black pepper, as required
- ¼ cup salt-free vegetable broth
- ¼ cup fresh cilantro, chopped

Instructions:

1. Preheat your oven to 375 °F. Lightly grease a large-sized baking dish.
2. In a large-sized bowl, add all ingredients except for cilantro and mix well.
3. Transfer the vegetable mixture into the prepared baking dish and then spread in an even layer.
4. Bake for approximately 15-20 minutes.
5. Serve immediately with the garnishing of cilantro.

Nutritional Information per Serving:

Calories: 96 - Fat: 5g - Sodium: 14mg - Carbohydrates: 13g - Fiber: 4.1g - Sugar: 7.9g - Protein: 1.9g

Veggies Casserole

Servings: 6 individuals
Preparation Time: 15 minutes
Cooking Time: 28 minutes

Ingredients:

For Onion Slices:

- ½ cup onion, very thinly sliced
- ¼ cup all-purpose white flour
- Freshly ground black pepper, as required

For Casserole:

- 1 pound fresh green beans, trimmed

- 1 tablespoon canola oil
- 8 ounces fresh cremini mushrooms, sliced
- ½ cup onion, thinly sliced
- 2 garlic cloves, minced
- Freshly ground black pepper, as required
- 1 tablespoon fresh thyme, chopped
- ½ cup salt-free vegetable broth
- ½ cup low-fat sour cream

Instructions:

1. Preheat your oven to 350 °F.
2. For onion slices: in a bowl, blend together all ingredients.
3. Place the onion mixture into a large-sized baking sheet in a single layer. Set aside.
4. Add green beans in a saucepan of boiling water and cook for approximately 5 minutes.
5. Drain and transfer into a bowl of ice water.
6. Drain well and transfer into a large-sized bowl.
7. In a large-sized wok, heat oil over medium-high heat and sauté mushrooms, onion, garlic and black pepper for approximately 2 minutes.
8. Stir in thyme and broth and cook for approximately 3-4 minutes or until all the liquid is absorbed.
9. Transfer the mushroom mixture into the bowl with green beans.
10. Add sour cream and stir to blend well.
11. Transfer the mixture into a 10-inch casserole dish.
12. Place casserole dish and baking sheet of onion slices into oven.
13. Bake for approximately 15-17 minutes.
14. Serve the casserole with the topping of crispy onion slices.

Nutritional Information per Serving:

Calories: 105 - Fat: 3.9g - Sodium: 24mg - Carbohydrates: 15.7g - Fiber: 3.6g - Sugar: 4.3g - Protein: 3.9g

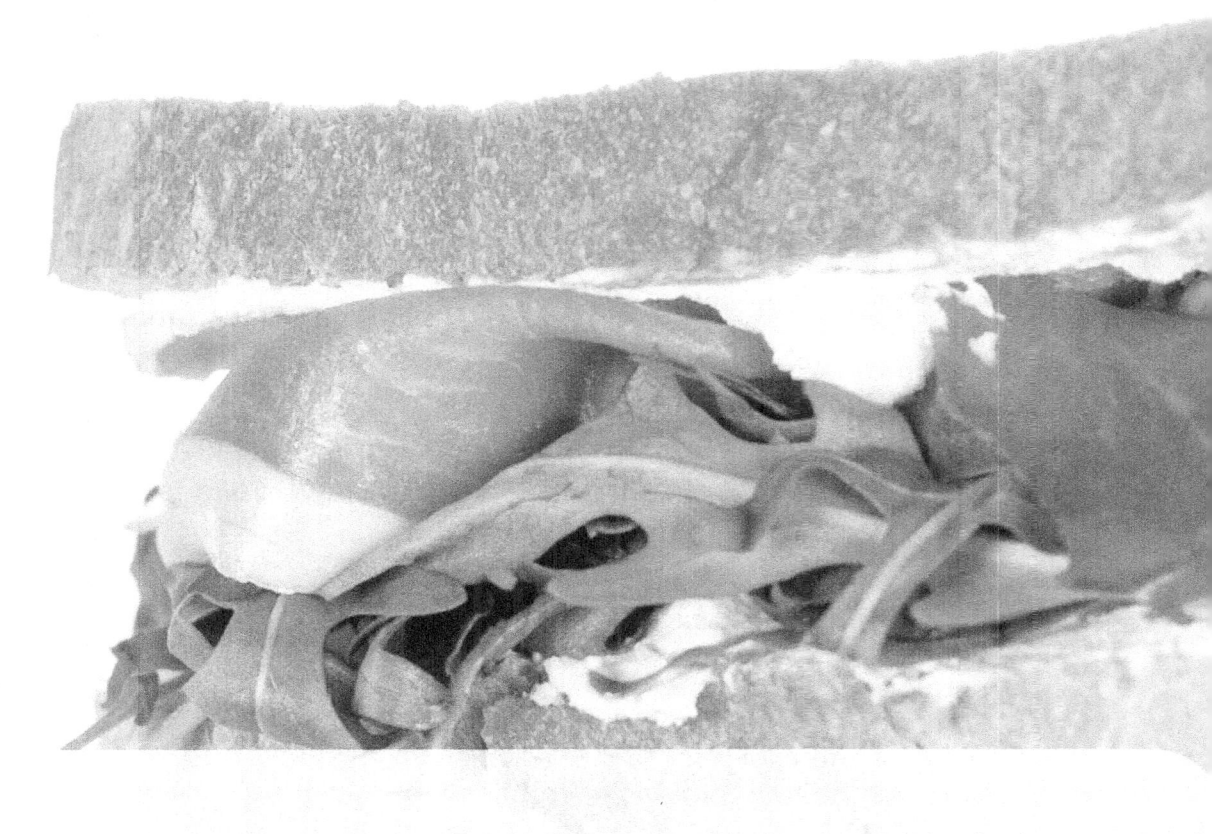

SNACKS
RECIPES

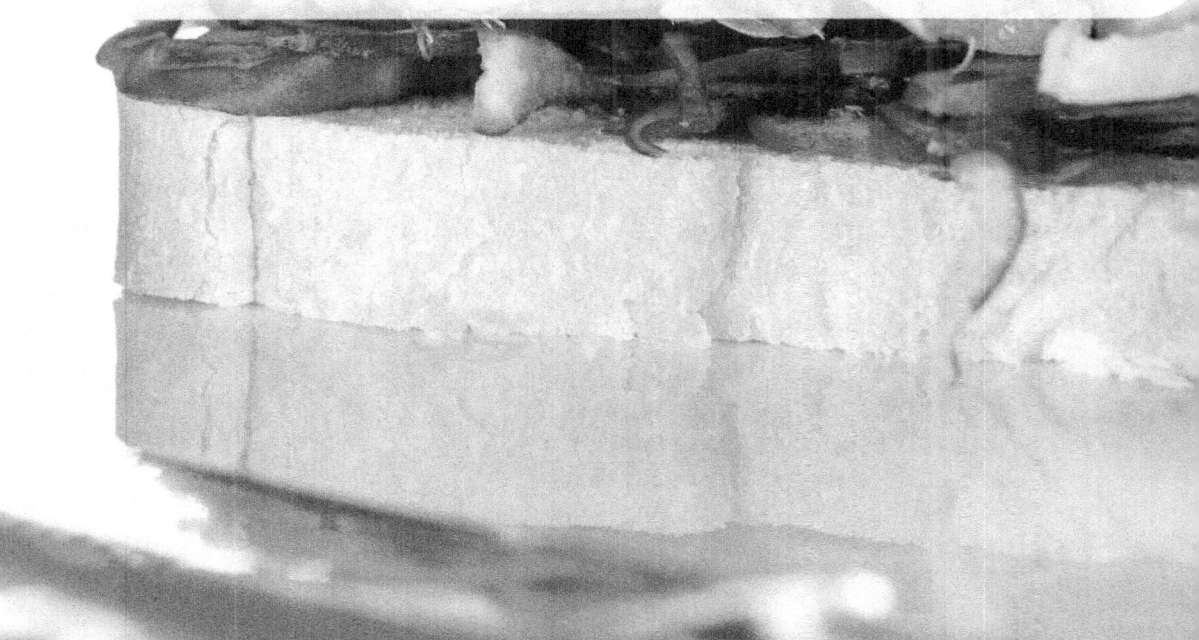

Grilled Watermelon

Servings: 4 individuals
Preparation Time: 10 minutes
Cooking Time: 4 minutes

Ingredients:

- Olive oil cooking spray
- 1 watermelon, peeled and cut into 1-inch thick wedges
- 1 garlic clove, minced finely
- 2 tablespoons fresh lime juice
- Pinch of cayenne powder

Instructions:

1. Preheat the grill to high heat.
2. Grease the grill grate with cooking spray.
3. Place the watermelon pieces onto the grill and cook for approximately 2 minutes from both sides.
4. Meanwhile, in a small-sized bowl, blend together the remaining ingredients.
5. Drizzle the watermelon slices with lemon mixture and serve.

Nutritional Information per Serving:

Calories: 11 - Fat: 0.1g - Sodium: 1mg -
Carbohydrates: 2.6g - Fiber: 0.2g -
Sugar: 1.9g - Protein: 0.2g

Apple Chips

Servings: 6 individuals
Preparation Time: 10 minutes
Cooking Time: 2 hours

Ingredients:

- 2 tablespoons ground cinnamon
- 1 tablespoon ground ginger
- 1½ teaspoons ground nutmeg
- 3 Fuji apples, sliced thinly in rounds

Instructions:

1. Preheat your oven to 200 ºF.
2. Line a baking sheet with parchment paper.
3. In a bowl, blend together all spices.
4. Arrange the apple slices into prepared baking sheet in a single layer and sprinkle with spice mixture generously.
5. Bake for approximately 1 hour.
6. Flip the side and again sprinkle with spice mixture.
7. Bake for approximately 1 hour.
8. Serve warm.

Nutritional Information per Serving:

Calories: 71 - Fat: 0.6g - Sodium: 3mg -
Carbohydrates: 18.5g - Fiber: 4.3g -
Sugar: 11.9g - Protein: 0.5g

Brussels Sprout Chips

Servings: 2 individuals
Preparation Time: 10 minutes
Cooking Time: 10 minutes

Ingredients:

- 2 cups Brussels sprout leaves (outer leaves)
- 2 tablespoons olive oil

Instructions:

1. Preheat your oven to 350 ºF.
2. Line two large-sized baking sheets with parchment paper.
3. Add Brussels sprout leaves and oil in a large-sized bowl and toss to coat well.
4. Divide the leaves onto the prepared baking sheets evenly and then spread in a single layer.
5. Bake for approximately 8-10 minutes or until crispy.
6. Serve immediately.

Nutritional Information per Serving:

Calories: 158 - Fat: 14.3g - Sodium: 22mg - Carbohydrates: 8g - Fiber: 3.3g - Sugar: 1.9g - Protein: 3g

Carrot Fries

Servings: 8 individuals
Preparation Time: 10 minutes
Cooking Time: 20 minutes

Ingredients:

- Olive oil cooking spray
- 6 large carrots, peeled and cut into 2-inch long sticks

Instructions:

1. Preheat your oven to 400 °F.
2. Lightly grease a large-sized baking sheet with cooking spray.
3. Place the carrot sticks onto the prepared baking sheet andthen arrange in a single layer.
4. Spray the carrot sticks with the cooking spray evenly.
5. Bake for approximately 20 minutes.
6. Serve hot.

Nutritional Information per Serving:

Calories: 22 - Fat: 0g - Sodium: 37mg - Carbohydrates: 5.3g - Fiber: 1.3g - Sugar: 2.7g - Protein: 0.4g

Cauliflower Poppers

Servings: 6 individuals
Preparation Time: 15 minutes
Cooking Time: 30 minutes

Ingredients:

- Olive oil cooking spray
- 4 cups cauliflower florets

- 2 teaspoons olive oil
- ¼ teaspoon red chili powder
- Freshly ground black pepper, as required

Instructions:

1. Preheat your oven to 450 °F.
2. Grease a roasting pan with cooking spray.
3. In a bowl, add all ingredients and toss to coat well.
4. Transfer the cauliflower mixture into the prepared roasting pan and spread in an even layer.
5. Roast for approximately 25-30 minutes.
6. Serve warm.

Nutritional Information per Serving:

Calories: 30 - Fat: 1.7g - Sodium: 21mg - Carbohydrates: 3.6g - Fiber: 1.7g - Sugar: 1.6g - Protein: 1.3g

Zucchini Fries

Servings: 4 individuals
Preparation Time: 15 minutes
Cooking Time: 25 minutes

Ingredients:

- 2 medium zucchinis, cut into slices
- 2 egg whites
- 1 cup low-fat Parmesan cheese, grated
- ½ teaspoon garlic powder
- ½ teaspoon cayenne powder

Instructions:

1. Preheat your oven to 425 °F.
2. Line two baking sheets with parchment paper.
3. In a small-sized shallow bowl, place the egg whites and whisk lightly.

4. In another medium-sized shallow dish, blend together the Parmesan and spices.
5. Dip the zucchini slices in the egg and then coat with Parmesan mixture.
6. Place the zucchini slices onto the prepared baking sheets and arrange in a single layer.
7. Bake for approximately 25-30 minutes, flipping once halfway through.
8. Serve hot.
9. Serve immediately.

Nutritional Information per Serving:

Calories: 29 - Fat: 0.3g - Sodium: 59mg - Carbohydrates: 4.3g - Fiber: 1.2g - Sugar: 1.9g - Protein: 3.3g

Chicken Nuggets

Servings: 8 individuals
Preparation Time: 15 minutes
Cooking Time: 30 minutes

Ingredients:

- 2 (8-ounce) skinless, boneless chicken breasts
- 4 egg whites
- 1 cup all-purpose white flour
- 1 teaspoon dried oregano, crushed
- ½ teaspoon paprika
- Freshly ground black pepper, as required

Instructions:

1. Preheat your oven to 350 ºF.
2. Cut each chicken breast into 2x1-inch chunks.
3. In a bowl, whisk the egg whites well.
4. Place the flour, oregano, paprika and black pepper in another shallow bowl and mix until well blended.

5. Dip the chicken nuggets in beaten eggs and then, evenly coat with the flour mixture.
6. Place the chicken chunks onto the prepared baking sheet and then arrange in a single layer.
7. Bake for approximately 30 minutes or until golden brown.
8. Serve warm.

Nutritional Information per Serving:

Calories: 137 - Fat: 2.2g - Sodium: 37mg - Carbohydrates: 12.3g - Fiber: 0.8g - Sugar: 0.2g - Protein: 16.1g

Cinnamon Popcorn

Servings: 3 individuals
Preparation Time: 10 minutes
Cooking Time: 5 minutes

Ingredients:

- 2 tablespoons unsalted butter
- ¾ cup popping corn
- ¼ teaspoon ground cinnamon

Instructions:

1. In a saucepan, melt butter over medium-high heat.
2. Add popping corn and cover the pan tightly.
3. Cook for approximately 1-2 minutes or until corn kernels start to pop, shaking the pan occasionally.
4. Remove the saucepan from heat and transfer into a large-sized heatproof bowl.
5. Add cinnamon and mix well.
6. Serve immediately

Nutritional Information per Serving:

Calories: 158 - Fat: 8.7g - Sodium: 55mg - Carbohydrates: 18.2g - Fiber: 4.1g - Sugar: 0g - Protein: 2.6g

Berries Gazpacho

Servings: 6 individuals
Preparation Time: 10 minutes

Ingredients:

- 2 cups fresh strawberries, hulled and sliced
- 2 cups fresh raspberries
- 4 cups fat-free milk
- ½ teaspoon organic vanilla extract

Instructions:

1. In a clean food processor, add berries, milk and vanilla extract and pulse until smooth.
2. Transfer the gazpacho into a large-sized serving bowl and refrigerate to chill before serving.

Nutritional Information per Serving:

Calories: 98 - Fat: 0.4g - Sodium: 88mg - Carbohydrates: 16.6g - Fiber: 3.6g - Sugar: 12.2g - Protein: 6.1g

Fruity Salsa

Servings: 8 individuals
Preparation Time: 15 minutes

Ingredients:

- 8 ounces fresh pineapple, chopped
- 2 large mangoes, peeled, pitted and chopped
- ½ cup red onion, chopped
- 1 tablespoon fresh ginger, grated finely
- ¼ cup fresh cilantro, chopped
- 1 teaspoon red pepper flakes
- 3 tablespoon apple cider vinegar

Instructions:

1. Add all ingredients in a large serving bowl and gently stir to blend.
2. Serve immediately.

Nutritional Information per Serving:

Calories: 72 - Fat: 0.4g - Sodium: 2mg - Carbohydrates: 17.7g - Fiber: 2.1g - Sugar: 17.7g - Protein: 1g

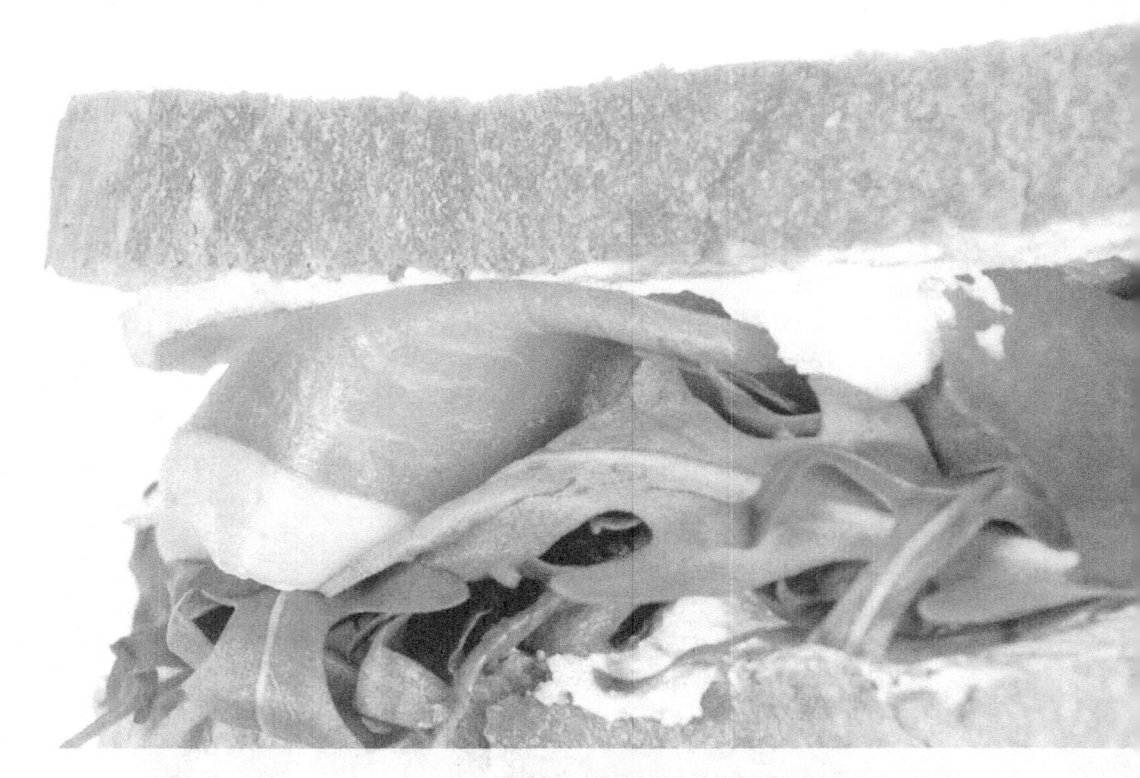

SANDWICHES & WRAPS

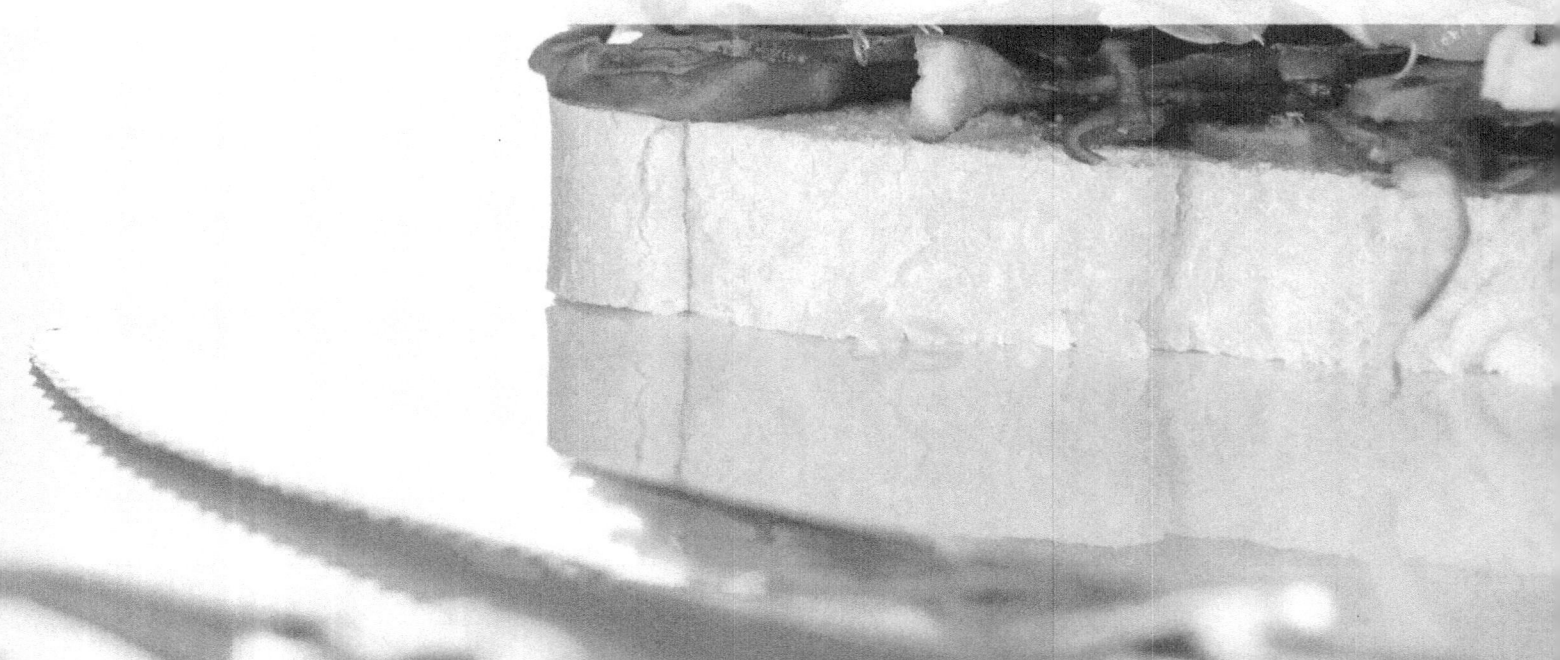

Chicken Lettuce Wraps

Servings: 2 individuals
Preparation Time: 15 minutes

Ingredients:

- 4 ounces unsalted cooked chicken, cut into strips
- ½ cup fresh strawberries, hulled and thinly sliced
- 1 small cucumber, thinly sliced
- 1 tablespoon fresh mint leaves, chopped
- 4 large lettuce leaves

Instructions:

1. In a large-sized bowl, add all ingredients except for lettuce leaves and gently toss to coat well.
2. Place the lettuce leaves onto serving plates.
3. Divide the chicken mixture over each leaf evenly.
4. Serve immediately.

Nutritional Information per Serving:

Calories: 122 - Fat: 2g - Sodium: 41mg - Carbohydrates: 8.8g - Fiber: 1.7g - Sugar: 4.4g - Protein: 17.8g

Shrimp Lettuce Wraps

Servings: 2 individuals
Preparation Time: 15 minutes
Cooking Time: 7 minutes

Ingredients:

- 1 tablespoon olive oil
- 1 garlic clove, minced
- 1 medium bell pepper, seeded and chopped
- 1/3 pound medium shrimp, peeled, deveined and chopped
- Freshly ground black pepper, as required

- 4 large lettuce leaves

Instructions:

1. Heat oil in a large-sized wok over medium heat and sauté garlic for approximately 30 seconds.
2. Add bell pepper and cook for approximately 2-3 minutes.
3. Add shrimp and black pepper and cook for approximately 2-3 minutes.
4. Remove from heat and cool slightly.
5. Divide the shrimp mixture over lettuce leaves evenly.
6. Serve immediately.

Nutritional Information per Serving:

Calories: 155 - Fat: 8.1g - Sodium: 124mg - Carbohydrates: 5.3g - Fiber: 0.9g - Sugar: 3.1g - Protein: 17g

Veggie Lettuce Wraps

Servings: 3 individuals
Preparation Time: 15 minutes

Ingredients:

- 1½ cups cucumber, chopped
- 1½ cups carrot, peeled and chopped
- 2 tablespoons scallions, chopped
- Freshly ground black pepper, as required
- 6 large lettuce leaves

Instructions:

1. Add the cucumber, carrot, scallion, and black pepper in a large bowl and mix well.
2. Arrange the lettuce leaves onto a smooth surface.
3. Divide the cucumber mixture onto each lettuce leaf evenly.
4. Serve immediately.

Nutritional Information per Serving:

Calories: 33 - Fat: 0.1g - Sodium: 40mg - Carbohydrates: 7.9g - Fiber: 1.8g - Sugar: 3.8g - Protein: 0.9g

Chicken & Mango Tortilla Wraps

Servings: 8 individuals
Preparation Time: 15 minutes

Ingredients:

- 2 tablespoons fresh lime juice
- 2 tablespoons olive oil
- Freshly ground black pepper, as required
- 2 cups unsalted cooked chicken, shredded
- 1 cup mango, peeled, pitted and cut into cubes
- 1 cup cabbage, shredded
- ¼ cup fresh cilantro, chopped
- 4 corn tortillas, warmed

Instructions:

1. In a large-sized bowl, add lime juice, oil and black pepper and whisk until well blended.
2. Add chicken, mango, cabbage and cilantro and toss to coat well.
3. Arrange the tortillas onto a smooth surface.
4. Place chicken mixture over each tortilla, leaving about 1-inch border all around.
5. Carefully fold the edges of each tortilla over the filling to roll up.
6. Cut each roll in half cross-wise and serve.

Nutritional Information per Serving:

Calories: 126 - Fat: 5.1g - Sodium: 132mg - Carbohydrates: 9.1g - Fiber: 1.4g - Sugar: 3.2g - Protein: 11.2g

Chicken & Veggie Tortilla Wraps

Servings: 8 individuals
Preparation Time: 15 minutes

Ingredients:

- ½ cup low-sodium mayonnaise
- 1 small garlic clove, finely minced
- 8 ounces unsalted cooked chicken, chopped
- 1 bell pepper, seeded and chopped
- 1 onion, chopped
- 4 corn tortillas, warmed

Instructions:

1. In a bowl, blend together mayonnaise and garlic.
2. In another bowl, blend together chicken and vegetables.
3. Arrange the tortillas onto a smooth surface.
4. Spread the mayonnaise mixture over each tortilla evenly.
5. Place chicken mixture over ¼ of each tortilla.
6. Fold the outside edges inward and roll up like a burrito.
7. Secure each tortilla with toothpicks.
8. Cut each tortilla in half and serve.

Nutritional Information per Serving:

Calories: 110 - Fat: 3.3g - Sodium: 154mg - Carbohydrates: 11.9g - Fiber: 1.3g - Sugar: 2.4g - Protein: 9.2g

Veggie Tortilla Wraps

Servings: 8 individuals
Preparation Time: 15 minutes
Cooking Time: 21 minutes

Ingredients:

- 1½ cups broccoli florets, chopped

- 1½ cups cauliflower florets, chopped
- 1 tablespoon water
- 2 teaspoons canola oil
- 1½ cups onion, chopped
- 1 garlic clove, minced
- 2 tablespoons fresh parsley, finely chopped
- 1 cup low-cholesterol liquid egg substitute
- Freshly ground black pepper, as required
- 4 corn tortillas, warmed

Instructions:

1. In a microwave-safe bowl, place broccoli, cauliflower and water and microwave, covered for approximately 3-5 minutes.
2. Remove from microwave and drain any liquid.
3. Heat canola oil in a wok over medium heat and sauté onion for approximately 4-5 minutes.
4. Add garlic and sauté for approximately 1 minute.
5. Stir in broccoli, cauliflower, parsley, egg substitute and black pepper.
6. Now, reduce the heat to medium-low and simmer for approximately 10 minutes.
7. Remove the wok of veggies from heat and set it aside to cool slightly.
8. Place broccoli mixture over ¼ of each tortilla.
9. Fold the outside edges inward and roll up like a burrito.
10. Secure the tortilla with toothpicks to secure the filling.
11. Cut each tortilla in half and serve.

Nutritional Information per Serving:

Calories: 73 - Fat: 1.6g - Sodium: 78mg - Carbohydrates: 9.9g - Fiber: 2.2g - Sugar: 2g - Protein: 5.6g

Chicken Sandwich

Servings: 4 individuals
Preparation Time: 15 minutes
Cooking Time: 16 minutes

Ingredients:

- Olive oil cooking spray
- ½ cup onion, sliced
- 1 garlic clove, minced
- 4 white bread slices
- ¼ cup low-fat cheddar cheese, shredded
- 2 lettuce leaves, torn
- ½ cup cooked chicken, shredded

Instructions:

1. Grease a non-stick wok with cooking spray and heat it over medium-low heat.
2. Add in onion and garlic and cook for approximately 10 minutes, stirring occasionally.
3. Arrange 2 bread slices onto a smooth surface.
4. Sprinkle about 2 tablespoons of cheese over each slice evenly.
5. Arrange lettuce over each slice, followed by onion mixture and chicken.
6. Sprinkle with remaining cheese evenly.
7. Cover with remaining 2 bread slices.
8. Again, grease the same non-stick wok with cooking spray and heat over medium heat.
9. Add the sandwiches and cook for approximately 3 minutes per side.
10. Cut each sandwich in half and serve.

Nutritional Information per Serving:

Calories: 86 - Fat: 3.2g - Sodium: 104mg - Carbohydrates: 6.3g - Fiber: 0.6g - Sugar: 1.1g - Protein: 7.7g

Turkey Sandwich

Servings: 4 individuals
Preparation Time: 15 minutes
Cooking Time: 4 minutes

Ingredients:

- 4 teaspoons low-sodium mayonnaise
- 4 white bread slices
- 1/3 cup unsalted cooked turkey, chopped
- 1 small apple, cored and thinly sliced
- 4 tablespoons part-skim mozzarella cheese, shredded
- 2 teaspoons olive oil

Instructions:

1. Spread mayonnaise over each slice evenly.
2. Place turkey over 2 slices, followed by apple slices and cheese.
3. Cover with remaining slices to make a sandwich.
4. Heat olive oil a large-sized non-stick frying pan over medium heat.
5. Place the sandwiches in frying pan and with a spoon, gently press down.
6. Cook for approximately 1-2 minutes.
7. Carefully flip the whole sandwich and cook for approximately 1-2 minutes.
8. Cut each sandwich in half and serve.

Nutritional Information per Serving:

Calories: 223 - Fat: 10.2g - Sodium: 184mg - Carbohydrates: 20.8g - Fiber: 2.1g - Sugar: 6.5g - Protein: 13.9g

Salmon Sandwich

Servings: 8 individuals
Preparation Time: 15 minutes
Cooking Time: 24 minutes

Ingredients:

- 8 white bread slices
- 1 cup low-fat Parmesan cheese, grated
- 12 ounces unsalted cooked salmon, chopped
- 2 tablespoons fresh dill, chopped finely
- 1 tablespoon fresh lemon zest, grated finely
- 2 tablespoons olive oil

Instructions:

1. Arrange 4 bread slices onto a smooth surface.
2. Place half of cheese over 4 slices, followed by salmon, dill, lemon zest and remaining cheese.
3. Cover with remaining bread slices to make sandwiches.
4. In a nonstick wok, heat ½ tablespoon of oil over medium heat.
5. Cook 1 sandwich for approximately 2-3 minutes per side.
6. Repeat with remaining oil and sandwiches.
7. Cut each sandwich in half and serve.

Nutritional Information per Serving:

Calories: 114 - Fat: 6.5g - Sodium: 94mg - Carbohydrates: 5.4g - Fiber: 0.4g - Sugar: 0.4g - Protein: 9.3g

Veggie Sandwich

Servings: 8 individuals
Preparation Time: 15 minutes

Ingredients:

- 1 large cucumber, sliced
- ½ cup onion, thinly sliced
- 1 cup romaine lettuce leaves, chopped
- ½ cup low-sodium mayonnaise
- 8 white bread slices, toasted

Instructions:

1. In a large-sized bowl, blend together cucumber, onion and lettuce.
2. Spread mayonnaise over each slice evenly.
3. Divide the lettuce mixture over 4 slices evenly.
4. Cover with remaining slices.
5. Cut each sandwich in half and serve.

Nutritional Information per Serving:

Calories: 118 - Fat: 5.8g - Sodium: 124mg - Carbohydrates: 15g - Fiber: 1.1g - Sugar: 1.7g - Protein: 2.6g

Drinks, Smoothies & Juices Recipes

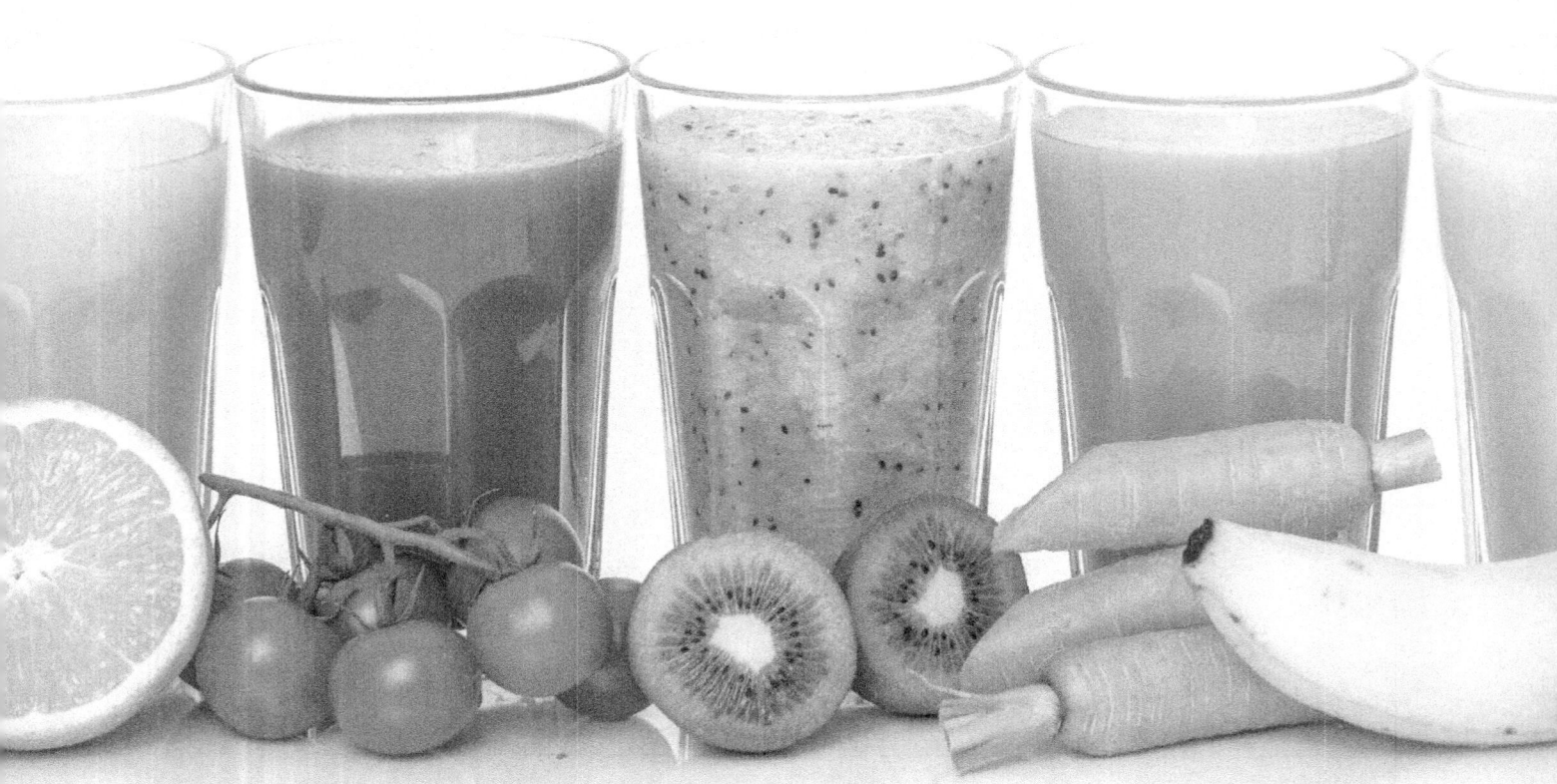

Citrus Detox Water

Servings: 3 individuals
Preparation Time: 10 minutes

Ingredients:

- 1 lime, cut into slices
- 1 lemon, cut into slices
- ½ of cucumber, cut into slices
- 2 tablespoons fresh mint leaves
- 6 cups filtered water

Instructions:

1. In a large-sized glass jar, place the orange, lime, lemon, cucumber and mint leaves and pour water on top.
2. Cover the jar with a lid and refrigerate for approximately 2-4 hours before serving.

Nutritional Information per Serving:

Calories: 13 - Fat: 0.1g - Sodium: 2mg - Carbohydrates: 3.4g - Fiber: 0.9g - Sugar: 1.1g - Protein: 0.6g

Lemonade

Servings: 4 individuals
Preparation Time: 10 minutes

Ingredients:

- ¾ cup fresh lemon juice
- 2-3 tablespoons honey
- 3½ cups cold water
- Ice cubes, as required

Instructions:

1. Add the lemon juice and honey in a large-sized pitcher and stir until dissolved.
2. Add the water and fill the pitcher with ice.
3. Serve chilled.

Nutritional Information per Serving:

Calories: 34 - Fat: 0.3g - Sodium: 8mg - Carbohydrates: 7.7g - Fiber: 4.6g - Sugar: 0.2g - Protein: 0.3g

Lemon Iced Tea

Servings: 6 individuals
Preparation Time: 10 minutes
Cooking Time: 5 minutes

Ingredients:

- 6 cups water
- ¼ cup fresh lemon juice
- 5 fresh thyme sprigs
- 1 cinnamon stick
- 3 black tea bags
- 3 teaspoons honey

Instructions:

1. In a large-sized saucepan, add water, lemon juice, thyme, lemon zest and cinnamon over medium-high heat and bring it to a boil.
2. Immediately remove the saucepan from heat and add in tea bags and honey.
3. Cover the pan and set aside for 15 minutes to steep.
4. Remove tea bags and thyme sprigs and let the tea cool for approximately an hour.
5. Through a fine mesh strainer, strain the tea mixture into a pitcher.
6. Refrigerate to chill before serving.

Nutritional Information per Serving:

Calories: 16 - Fat: 0.2g - Sodium: 3mg - Carbohydrates: 3.7g - Fiber: 0.4g - Sugar: 3.1g - Protein: 0.2g

Chilled Green Tea

Servings: 2 individuals
Preparation Time: 10 minutes

Ingredients:

- 2½ cups boiling water
- 1 cup fresh mint leaves
- 3 green tea bags
- 2 teaspoons honey

Instructions:

1. In a pitcher, blend together water, mint and tea bags.
2. Cover and steep for approximately 5 minutes.
3. Refrigerate for at least 3 hours.
4. Discard the tea bags and divide the tea in serving glasses.
5. Stir in honey and serve.

Nutritional Information per Serving:

Calories: 41 - Fat: 0.3g - Sodium: 14mg - Carbohydrates: 9.6g - Fiber: 3.1g - Sugar: 5.8g - Protein: 1.5g

Spiced Ginger Tea

Servings: 8 individuals
Preparation Time: 10 minutes
Cooking Time: 15 minutes

Ingredients:

- 10 cups water
- 1 (4-inch) piece fresh ginger, chopped
- 4 lemons, sliced
- 6 cardamom pods, bruised
- 1 cinnamon stick
- 1 whole star anise pod
- 4 tablespoons raw honey

Instructions:

1. In a saucepan, add water over medium-high heat and bring it to a boil.
2. Stir in ginger, lemon slices and spices and adjust the heat to medium-low.
3. Simmer for approximately 5-10 minutes.
4. Strain the tea into a pitcher.
5. Stir in honey and serve.

Nutritional Information per Serving:

Calories: 37 - Fat: 0.1g - Sodium: 1mg - Carbohydrates: 10.3g - Fiber: 0.7g - Sugar: 8.9g - Protein: 0.2g

Apple Smoothie

Servings: 2 individuals
Preparation Time: 10 minutes

Ingredients:

- 2 large apples, peeled, cored and chopped
- 2 teaspoons white sugar
- ½ cup fat-free plain Greek yogurt
- 1 cup fat-free milk
- ½ cup ice cubes

Instructions:

1. Add all the ingredients in a high-power blender and pulse until creamy.
2. Transfer the smoothie into glasses and serve immediately.

Nutritional Information per Serving:

Calories: 211 - Fat: 0.5g - Sodium: 54mg - Carbohydrates: 43.3g - Fiber: 5.4g - Sugar: 35.5g - Protein: 10.6g

Papaya Smoothie

Servings: 2 individuals
Preparation Time: 10 minutes

Ingredients:

- 2 cups papaya, peeled and sliced
- 1 teaspoon white sugar
- 1½ cups fat-free milk
- ¼ cup ice cubes

Instructions:

1. Add all the ingredients in a high-power blender and pulse until creamy.
2. Transfer the smoothie into glasses and serve immediately.

Nutritional Information per Serving:

Calories: 137 - Fat: 0.4g - Sodium: 94mg - Carbohydrates: 26.7g - Fiber: 2.5g - Sugar: 22.3g - Protein: 6.7g

Cranberry Smoothie

Servings: 2 individuals
Preparation Time: 10 minutes

Ingredients:

- 2 cups fresh cranberries
- 1 scoop unsweetened protein powder
- 2 teaspoons white sugar
- 1½ cups fat-free milk
- ¼ cup ice cubes

Instructions:

1. Add all the ingredients in a high-power blender and pulse until creamy.
2. Transfer the smoothie into glasses and serve immediately.

Nutritional Information per Serving:

Calories: 201 - Fat: 0.5g - Sodium: 124mg - Carbohydrates: 23g - Fiber: 4g - Sugar: 17g - Protein: 18.7g

Strawberry Smoothie

Servings: 2 individuals
Preparation Time: 10 minutes

Ingredients:

- 2 cups fresh strawberries, hulled and sliced
- 2 teaspoons white sugar
- 1½ cups fat-free milk
- ¼ cup ice cubes

Instructions:

1. Add all the ingredients in a high-power blender and pulse until creamy.
2. Transfer the smoothie into glasses and serve immediately.

Nutritional Information per Serving:

Calories: 129 - Fat: 0.4g - Sodium: 84mg - Carbohydrates: 24.1g - Fiber: 2.9g - Sugar: 20.1g - Protein: 7g

Raspberry Smoothie

Servings: 2 individuals
Preparation Time: 10 minutes

Ingredients:

- 2 cups fresh raspberries
- 1 scoop unflavored protein powder
- 2 teaspoons white sugar
- 1½ cups fat-free milk
- ¼ cup ice cubes

RENAL DIET COOKBOOK FOR BEGINNERS

Instructions:

1. Add all the ingredients in a high-power blender and pulse until creamy.
2. Transfer the smoothie into glasses and serve immediately.

Nutritional Information per Serving:

Calories: 200 - Fat: 1.6g - Sodium: 124mg - Carbohydrates: 27.7g - Fiber: 9g - Sugar: 18.4g - Protein: 20g

Strawberry Juice

Servings: 2 individuals
Preparation Time: 10 minutes

Ingredients:

- 2 cups fresh strawberries, hulled
- 1 teaspoon fresh lime juice
- 2 cups filtered water
- Ice cubes, as required

Instructions:

1. Place the strawberries, lime juice and water in a high-power blender and pulse until smooth.
2. Divide the ice cubes into two glasses.
3. Through a fine mesh strainer, strain the juice and transfer it into glasses over ice.
4. Serve immediately.

Nutritional Information per Serving:

Calories: 118 - Fat: 0.8g - Sodium: 3mg - Carbohydrates: 30.1g - Fiber: 6.5g - Sugar: 20.6g - Protein: 1.6g

Cranberry Juice

Servings: 2 individuals
Preparation Time: 10 minutes

Ingredients:

- 2 cups fresh cranberries
- 1 cup filtered water
- ½ tablespoon fresh lemon juice
- 2-3 tablespoons honey
- Ice cubes, as required

Instructions:

1. Place the cranberries, water, lemon juice and honey in a high-power blender and pulse until smooth.
2. Divide the ice cubes into two glasses.
3. Through a fine mesh strainer, strain the juice and transfer it into glasses over ice.
4. Serve immediately.

Nutritional Information per Serving:

Calories: 125 - Fat: 0g - Sodium: 2mg - Carbohydrates: 27.4g - Fiber: 4.1g - Sugar: 21.3g - Protein: 0.1g

Grapes Juice

Servings: 2 individuals
Preparation Time: 10 minutes

Ingredients:

- 2 cups seedless red grapes
- ½ lime, peel removed
- 2 cups filtered water
- Ice cubes, as required

Instructions:

1. Place the grapes, lime and water in a high-power blender and pulse until smooth.

2. Divide the ice cubes into two glasses.
3. Through a fine mesh strainer, strain the juice and transfer it into glasses over ice.
4. Serve immediately.

Nutritional Information per Serving:

Calories: 106 - Fat: 0g - Sodium: 3mg - Carbohydrates: 27.5g - Fiber: 1.1g - Sugar: 23.1g - Protein: 1g

Apple Juice

Servings: 2 individuals
Preparation Time: 10 minutes

Ingredients:

- 6 medium granny smith apples, cored and sliced
- 1 tablespoon fresh lime juice

Instructions:

1. Add apple slices into a juicer and extract the juice according to manufacturer's directions.
2. Stir in lemon juice and serve.

Nutritional Information per Serving:

Calories: 241 - Fat: 0g - Sodium: 0mg - Carbohydrates: 66.1g - Fiber: 15g - Sugar: 51g - Protein: 0g

Carrot Juice

Servings: 2 individuals
Preparation Time: 10 minutes

Ingredients:

- 8 large carrots, trimmed, peeled and cut into large chunks
- Pinch of ground black pepper

Instructions:

1. Place the carrots into a juicer and extract the juice according to the manufacturer's method.
2. Pour the juice into glasses and stir in black pepper.
3. Serve immediately.

Nutritional Information per Serving:

Calories: 100 - Fat: 0g - Sodium: 84mg - Carbohydrates: 24g - Fiber: 6g - Sugar: 12g - Protein: 2g

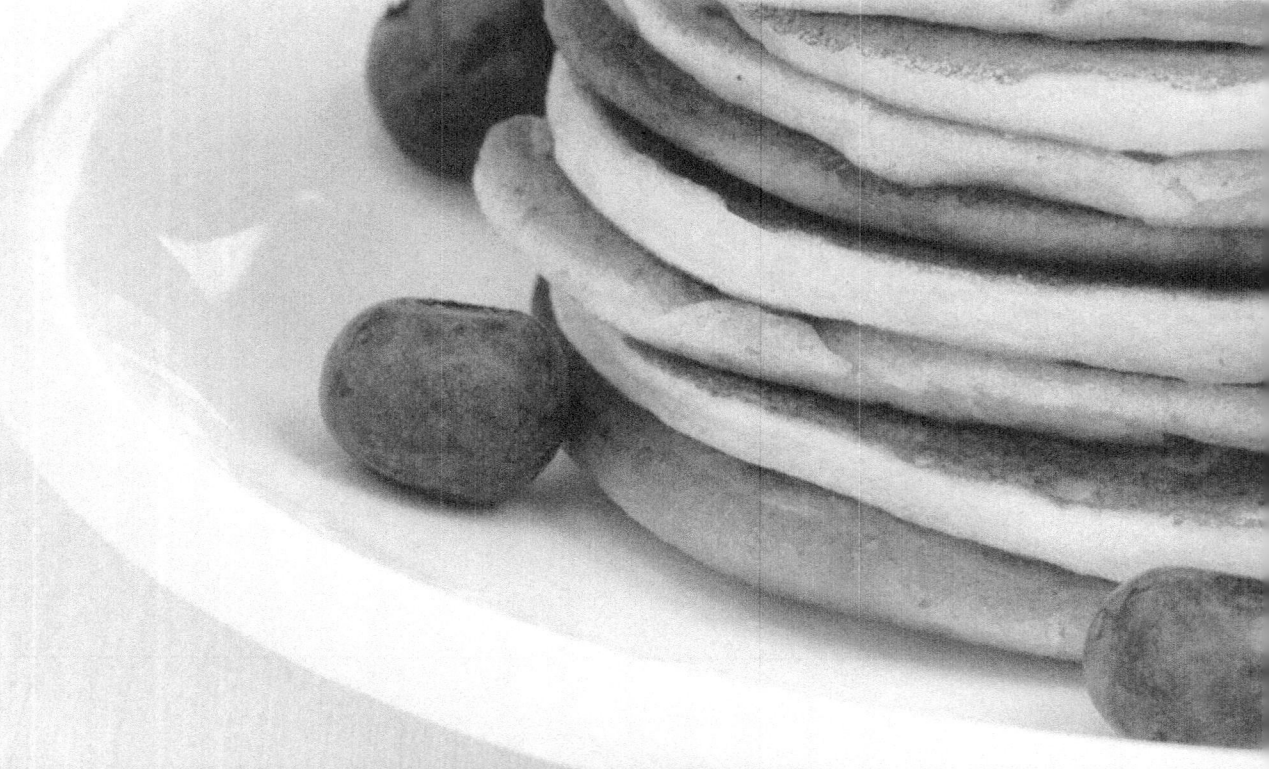

DESSERT

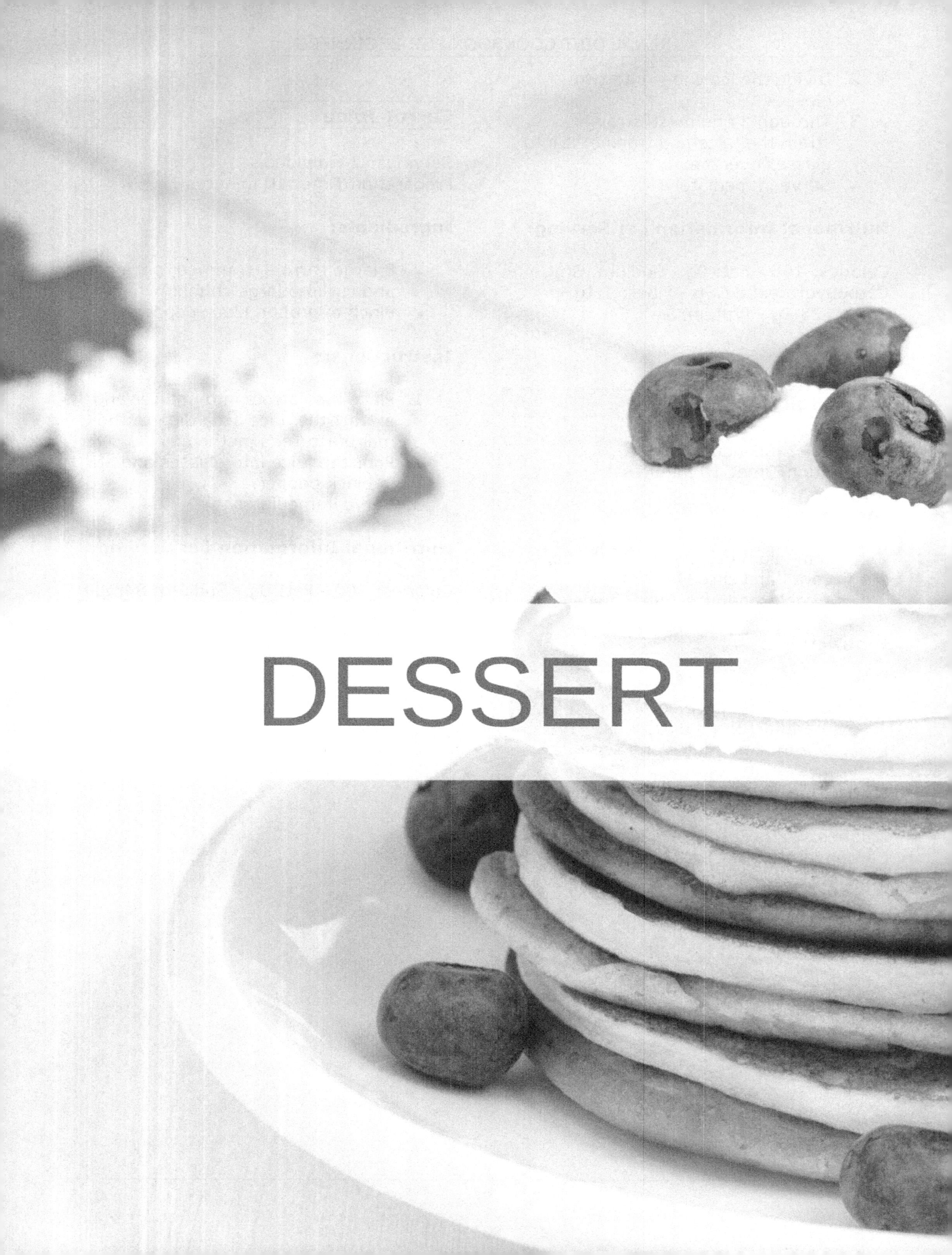

Baked Apples

Servings: 4 individuals
Preparation Time: 10 minutes
Cooking Time: 18 minutes

Ingredients:

- 4 small apples, cored
- 2 tablespoons unsalted butter, softened
- 2 teaspoons ground cinnamon
- 1/8 teaspoon ground ginger
- 1/8 teaspoon ground nutmeg

Instructions:

1. Preheat your oven to 350 °F.
2. Fill each apple with ½ tablespoon of butter.
3. Sprinkle each with spices evenly.
4. Arrange the apples onto a baking sheet.
5. Bake for approximately 12-18 minutes.
6. Serve warm.

Nutritional Information per Serving:

Calories: 170 - Fat: 6.2g - Sodium: 43mg - Carbohydrates: 31.8g - Fiber: 6g - Sugar: 23.2g - Protein: 07g

Strawberry Granita

Servings: 4 individuals
Preparation Time: 15 minutes

Ingredients:

- 2 cups fresh strawberries, hulled and sliced
- 1 tablespoon honey
- 1 tablespoon fresh lime juice
- 1 cup ice, crushed

Instructions:

1. In a high-powered blender, add the strawberries, honey, lemon juice and ice cubes and pulse on high speed until smooth.
2. Transfer the berry mixture into an 8x8-inch baking dish, spread evenly, and freeze for at least 30 minutes.
3. Remove from the freezer and, with a fork, stir the granita completely.
4. Freeze the baking dish of granita for 2-3 hours, stirring every 30 minutes with a fork.

Nutritional Information per Serving:

Calories: 39 - Fat: 0.2g - Sodium: 3mg - Carbohydrates: 9.9g - Fiber: 1.5g - Sugar: 7.8g - Protein: 2.5g

Lime Sorbet

Servings: 4 individuals
Preparation Time: 10 minutes

Ingredients:

- 2 tablespoons fresh lime zest, grated
- ½ cup maple syrup
- 2 cups water
- 1½ cups fresh lime juice

Instructions:

1. Freeze ice cream maker tub for approximately 24 hours before making this sorbet.
2. In a non-stick saucepan, add all of the ingredients except for lime juice over medium heat and cook for approximately 1 minute, stirring continuously.
3. Remove the pan of mixture from heat and stir in the lime juice.
4. Transfer this into an airtight container and refrigerate for approximately 2 hours.

5. Now, place the lime mixture into the ice cream maker and process it according to the manufacturer's directions.
6. Return the ice cream to the airtight container and freeze for approximately 2 hours.

Nutritional Information per Serving:

Calories: 130 - Fat: 0g - Sodium: 0mg - Carbohydrates: 33.4g - Fiber: 2.3g - Sugar: 30.2g - Protein: 0.1g

Strawberry Sundae

Servings: 2 individuals
Preparation Time: 10 minutes

Ingredients:

- ½ cup ricotta cheese
- 1 teaspoon organic vanilla extract
- 1 teaspoon fresh lemon juice
- 2-3 teaspoons powdered sugar
- ½ cup fresh strawberries, hulled and sliced

Instructions:

1. Add all the ingredients except strawberries in a medium-sized bowl and whisk until smooth.
2. In a serving glass, place half of cheese mixture.
3. Place strawberries over cheese mixture.
4. Top with remaining cheese mixture and serve immediately.

Nutritional Information per Serving:

Calories: 113 - Fat: 5g - Sodium: 74mg - Carbohydrates: 25.4g - Fiber: 8.8g - Sugar: 4.7g - Protein: 7.3g

Raspberry Pudding

Servings: 4 individuals
Preparation Time: 10 minutes

Ingredients:

- 2½ cups fresh raspberries
- 1/3 cup white sugar
- 1/3 cup unsweetened rice milk
- 1 tablespoon fresh lemon juice

Instructions:

1. Add all the ingredients and pulse until smooth in a clean food processor.
2. Transfer the mixture into serving glasses and refrigerate to chill before serving.

Nutritional Information per Serving:

Calories: 107 - Fat: 0.8g - Sodium: 17mg - Carbohydrates: 26.1g - Fiber: 5.1g - Sugar: 20.2g - Protein: 1g

Raspberry Jelly

Servings: 4 individuals
Preparation Time: 10 minutes
Cooking Time: 40 minutes

Ingredients:

- 2 pounds fresh raspberries
- ¼ cup water
- 1 tablespoon fresh lemon juice

Instructions:

1. In a medium-sized saucepan, add the raspberries and water and cook over low heat for 8-10 minutes or until raspberries become soft, stirring occasionally.
2. Add the lemon juice and cook for 30 minutes.

3. Remove from heat and place the mixture into a sieve.
4. Strain the mixture into a bowl by pressing with the back of a spoon.
5. Now, transfer the mixture into a blender and pulse until a jelly like texture is formed.
6. Transfer into glass serving bowls and refrigerate for 1-2 hours before serving.

Nutritional Information per Serving:

Calories: 119 - Fat: 1.5g - Sodium: 3mg - Carbohydrates: 27.2g - Fiber: 14.8g - Sugar: 10.1g - Protein: 2.8g

Strawberry Soufflé

Servings: 6 individuals
Preparation Time: 10 minutes
Cooking Time: 10 minutes

Ingredients:

- 18 ounces fresh strawberries, hulled
- 1/3 cup honey, divided
- 5 egg whites, divided
- 4 teaspoons fresh lemon juice

Instructions:

1. Preheat your oven to 350 ºF.
2. In a high-powered blender, add strawberries and pulse until a puree forms.
3. Through a strainer, strain the seeds.
4. In a large-sized bowl, add strawberry puree, 3 tablespoons of honey, 2 egg whites and lemon juice and pulse until frothy and light.
5. In another bowl, add remaining egg whites and whisk until frothy.
6. While beating gradually, add remaining honey and whisk until stiff peaks form.
7. Gently fold the egg whites into strawberry mixture.

8. Transfer the mixture into 6 large ramekins evenly.
9. Arrange the ramekins onto a baking sheet.
10. Bake for approximately 10-12 minutes.
11. Serve immediately.

Nutritional Information per Serving:

Calories: 100 - Fat: 0.3g - Sodium: 30mg - Carbohydrates: 22.3c - Fiber: 1.8g - Sugar: 19.8g - Protein: 3.7g

Strawberry Muffins

Servings: 8 individuals
Preparation Time: 15 minutes
Cooking Time: 25 minutes

Ingredients:

- 1 cup buckwheat flour
- ¼ cup arrowroot starch
- 1½ teaspoons baking powder
- 4 egg whites
- ½ cup fat-free milk
- 2-3 tablespoons maple syrup
- 2 tablespoons unsalted butter, melted
- 1 cup fresh strawberries, hulled and chopped

Instructions:

1. Preheat your oven to 350 ºF. Line 8 cups of a muffin tin.
2. In a medium-sized bowl, mix the buckwheat flour, arrowroot starch and baking powder.
3. In a separate glass bowl, place the eggs, milk, maple syrup and butter and whisk until well blended.
4. Now, place the flour mixture and mix until just combined.
5. Gently fold in the strawberry pieces.
6. Transfer the mixture into prepared muffin cups evenly.
7. Bake for approximately 25 minutes.

8. Remove the muffin tin from oven and place onto a wire rack to cool for approximately 10 minutes.
9. Then invert the muffins onto the wire rack to cool completely before serving.

Nutritional Information per Serving:

Calories: 123 - Fat: 3.4g - Sodium: 48mg - Carbohydrates: 20.1g - Fiber: 2g - Sugar: 5.1g - Protein: 4.3g

Blueberry Muffins

Servings: 12 individuals
Preparation Time: 15 minutes
Cooking Time: 25 minutes

Ingredients:

- Olive oil cooking spray
- 2 cups all-purpose white flour
- ½ cup white sugar
- 2 teaspoons baking powder
- 1 cup unsweetened rice milk
- 2 large egg whites, lightly beaten
- ¼ cup canola oil
- 1 cup frozen blueberries
- 1 tablespoon lemon zest, finely grated

Instructions:

1. Preheat your oven to 375 °F.
2. Lightly grease a 12 cups muffin pan with cooking spray.
3. In a bowl, blend together flour, sugar and baking powder.
4. In another bowl, add rice milk, egg whites and oil and whisk until well blended.
5. Add egg mixture into flour mixture and mix until just moistened.
6. Gently fold in blueberries and lemon zest.
7. Place the mixture into prepared muffin cups evenly.
8. Bake for approximately 25 minutes.

9. Remove the muffin tin from oven and place onto a wire rack to cool for approximately 10 minutes.
10. Then invert the muffins onto the wire rack to cool completely before serving.

Nutritional Information per Serving:

Calories: 162 - Fat: 5g - Sodium: 18mg - Carbohydrates: 27.3g - Fiber: 1.4g - Sugar: 9.7g - Protein: 2.9g

Bread Casserole

Servings: 8 individuals
Preparation Time: 10 minutes
Cooking Time: 6 minutes

Ingredients:

- 1¼ cups fat-free milk
- 8 egg whites
- 4 (¾-inch thick) white bread slices, trimmed and diagonally sliced
- 2 tablespoons olive oil
- 3 tablespoons sugar-free syrup

Instructions:

1. Preheat your oven to 400 °F.
2. Arrange a baking sheet in the oven to heat.
3. In a bowl, add milk and eggs and whisk slightly.
4. Dip each bread slice in egg mixture evenly.
5. In a large-sized, non-stick wok, heat olive oil over medium heat and cook the bread slices for approximately 1 minute per side.
6. Now, arrange the slices onto hot baking sheet in a single layer.
7. Bake for approximately 4 minutes.
8. Drizzle with syrup and serve.

Nutritional Information per Serving:

Calories: 93 - Fat: 3.9g - Sodium: 124mg - Carbohydrates: 8.8g - Fiber: 0.4g - Sugar: 2.5g - Protein: 6g

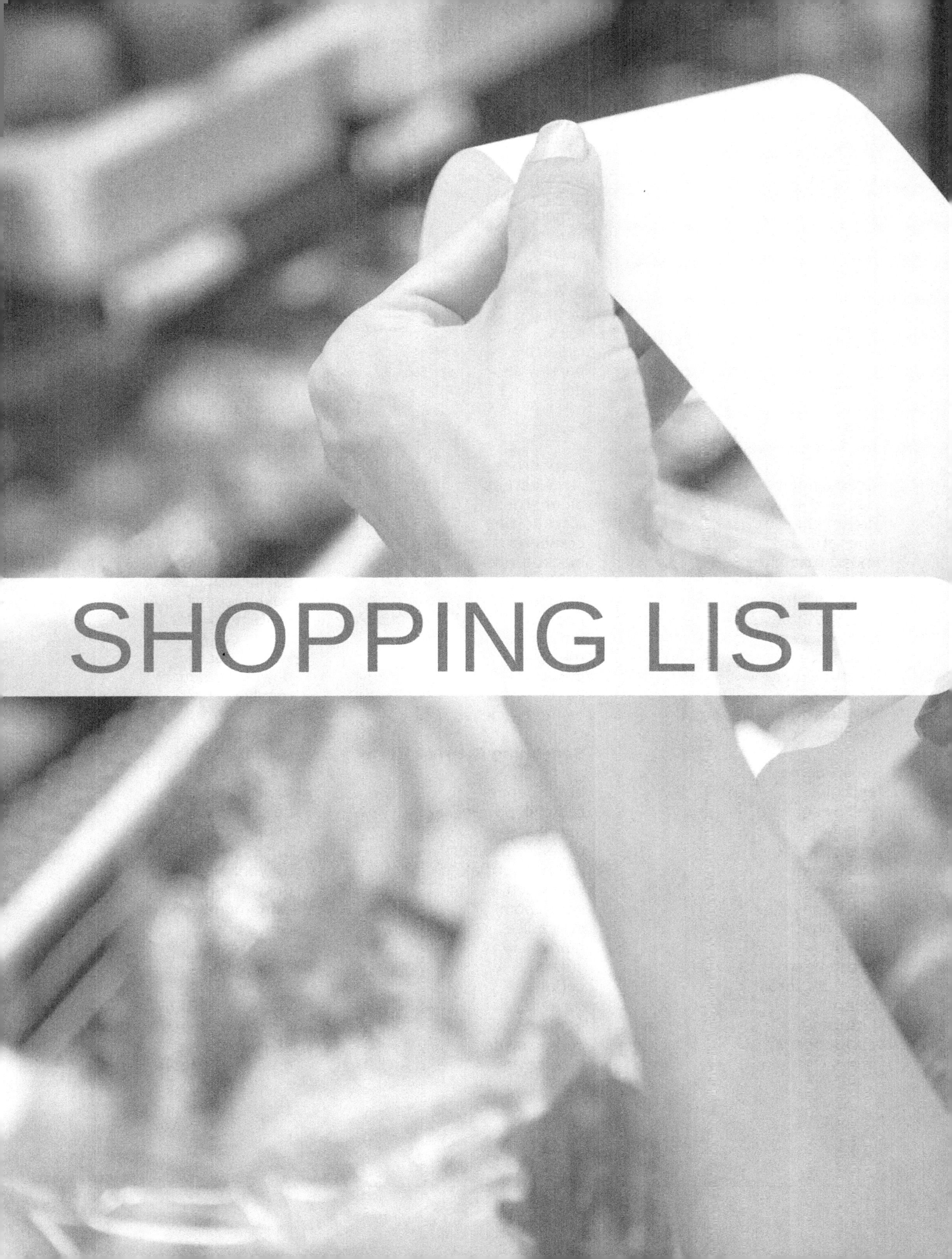

SHOPPING LIST

Poultry, Meat & Seafood

chicken breasts
chicken thighs
chicken tenders
cooked chicken
ground chicken
ground turkey
cooked turkey
beef chuck roast
ground beef
salmon
cod
shrimp
scallops

Dairy:

eggs
fat-free milk
butter
Greek yogurt
half-and-half creamer
cream cheese
sour cream
mozzarella cheese
Parmesan cheese
cheddar cheese
cottage cheese
goat cheese
feta cheese
ricotta cheese

Vegetables & Fresh Herbs:

mushrooms
zucchini
yellow squash
eggplant
broccoli
cauliflower
cabbage
bell pepper
asparagus
carrot
green beans
Brussels sprout
celery
lettuce
cucumber
onion

shallot
scallion
ginger
garlic
green chili
Serrano pepper
jalapeño pepper
lemon
lime
chives
oregano
thyme
basil
mint
cilantro
parsley
dill

Fruit

raspberries
strawberries
blueberries
blackberries
cranberries
blackberries
watermelon
grapes
papaya
pineapple
mango
apple
pear
canned peaches

Seasoning & Dried Herbs

black pepper
red chili powder
paprika
cayenne powder
red pepper flakes
cinnamon
cardamom
star anise
ginger
cumin
coriander
turmeric
garlic powder
curry powder
bay leaves

dill
oregano
thyme
basil

Extra:

margarine
olive oil
canola oil
cooking spray
rice milk
all-purpose white flour
oat flour
cornmeal
arrowroot powder
arrowroot starch
cornstarch
quinoa
buckwheat
oats
popping corn
Arborio rice
white rice
buckwheat noodles
wheat berries
baking powder
baking soda
protein powder
active dry yeast
white sugar
powdered sugar
maple syrup
honey
applesauce
pancake syrup
sugar-free syrup
vanilla extract
balsamic vinegar
apple cider vinegar
BBQ sauce
mayonnaise
unsweetened coconut
cinnamon bread
white bread
pita breads
corn tortillas
chicken broth
vegetable broth
liquid egg substitute
black tea bags
green tea bags

28-Day
Meal Plan

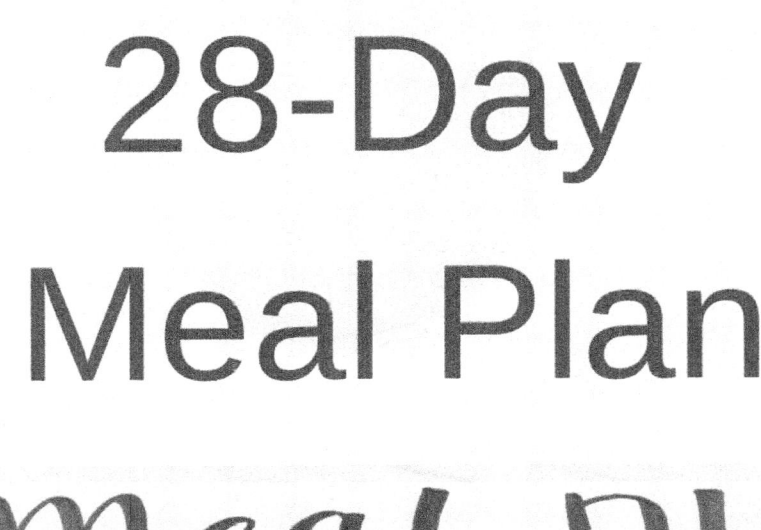

Meal Plan		
Sun		
Mon		
Tue		
Wed		
Thu		
Fri		
Sat		

Day 1:

Breakfast: Blueberry Bread

Lunch: Shrimp & Watermelon Kabobs

Dinner: Salmon & Shrimp Stew

Day 2:

Breakfast: Apple Omelet

Lunch: Zucchini Noodles with Mushroom Sauce

Dinner: Salmon in Yogurt Sauce

Day 3:

Breakfast: Berries Cheese & Yogurt Bowl

Lunch: Lemony Shrimp

Dinner: Veggies Casserole

Day 4:

Breakfast: Cottage Cheese Pancakes

Lunch: Stuffed Zucchini

Dinner:

Day 5:

Breakfast: Raspberry Smoothie Bowl

Lunch: Cauliflower Soup

Dinner: Cod & Mushroom Casserole

Day 6:

Breakfast: Zucchini Omelet

Lunch: Mixed Fruit Salad

Dinner: Baked Beef Stew

Day 7:

Breakfast: Fruity Wheat Berries Bowl

Lunch: Chicken Pita Pizza

Dinner: Curried Veggies Bake

Day 8:

Breakfast: Chives Waffles

Lunch: Stuffed Bell Peppers

Dinner: Turkey & Zucchini Chili

Day 9:

Breakfast: Cheese & Egg Whites Scramble

Lunch: Veggie Tortilla Wraps

Dinner: Beef Casserole

Day 10:

Breakfast: Cauliflower & Pear Porridge

Lunch: Asparagus Risotto

Dinner: Chicken with Veggies

Day 11:

Breakfast: Apple Smoothie

Lunch: Chicken Meatballs

Dinner: Veggies Casserole

Day 12:

Breakfast: Zucchini Frittata

Lunch: Asparagus Soup

Dinner: Chicken in Dill Sauce

Day 13:

Breakfast: Vanilla Pancakes

Lunch: Scallops in Garlic Sauce

Dinner: Curried Veggies Bake

Day 14:

Breakfast: Zucchini Muffins

Lunch: Papaya & Carrot Salad

Dinner: Chicken & Cauliflower Stew

Day 15:

Breakfast: Fruity Yogurt Bowl

Lunch: Veggie Sandwich

Dinner: Chicken & Berries Salad

Day 16:

Breakfast: Blueberry Bread

Lunch: Salmon Burgers

Dinner: Baked Beef Stew

Day 17:

Breakfast: Apple Strata

Lunch: Veggie Lettuce Wraps

Dinner: Chicken with Veggies

Day 18:

Breakfast: Cornmeal Waffles

Lunch: Chicken Pita Pizza

Dinner: Shrimp & Veggie Salad

Day 19:

Breakfast: Chicken Muffins

Lunch: Buckwheat Noodles with Mushrooms

Dinner: Salmon Soup

Day 20:

Breakfast: Cauliflower & Pear Porridge

Lunch: Chicken & Mango Tortilla Wraps

Dinner: Curried Veggies Bake

Day 21:

Breakfast: Strawberry Smoothie

Lunch: Shrimp & Watermelon Kabobs

Dinner: Ground Turkey & Cabbage Soup

Day 22:

Breakfast: Microwave Egg Whites Scramble

Lunch: Asparagus Soup

Dinner: Salmon & Cucumber Salad

Day 23:

Breakfast: Raspberry Smoothie Bowl

Lunch: Chicken & Pineapple Kabobs

Dinner: Veggie Casserole

Day 24:

Breakfast: Yogurt Oatmeal

Lunch: Watermelon & Cucumber Salad

Dinner: Chicken & Cabbage Soup

Day 25:

Breakfast: Apple Strata

Lunch: Chicken Lettuce Wraps

Dinner: Salmon & Shrimp Stew

Day 26:

Breakfast: Quinoa Bread

Lunch: Stuffed Zucchini

Dinner: Ground Turkey with Veggies

Day 27:

Breakfast: Cornmeal Waffles

Lunch: Beef & Veggie Meatballs

Dinner: Chicken with Veggies

Day 28:

Breakfast: Chicken Muffins

Lunch: Asparagus Risotto

Dinner: Shrimp & Veggie Salad

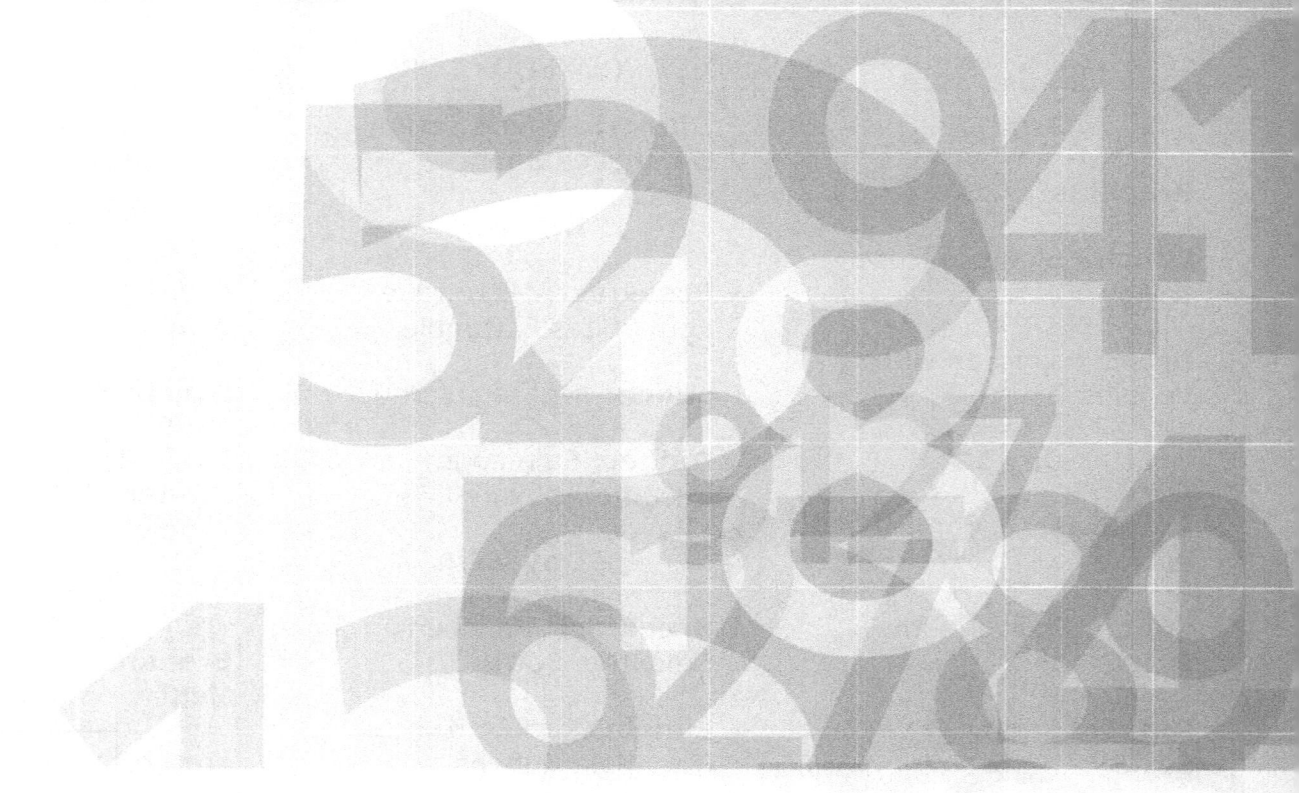

CONVERSION TABLES

MASS

Imperial (ounces)	Metric (gram)
¼ ounce	7 grams
½ ounce	14 grams
1 ounce	28 grams
2 ounces	56 grams
3 ounces	85 grams
4 ounces	113 grams
5 ounces	141 grams
6 ounces	150 grams
7 ounces	198 grams
8 ounces	226 grams
9 ounces	255 grams
10 ounces	283 grams
11 ounces	311 grams
12 ounces	340 grams
13 ounces	368 grams
14 ounces	396 grams
15 ounces	425 grams
16 ounces/ 1 pound	455 grams

CUPS & SPOON

Cups	Metric
¼ cup	60 milliliters
1/3 cup	80 milliliters
½ cup	120 milliliters
1 cup	240 milliliters
Spoon	Metric
¼ teaspoon	1¼ milliliters
½ teaspoon	2½ milliliters
1 teaspoon	5 milliliters
2 teaspoons	10 milliliters
1 tablespoon	30 milliliters

LIQUID

Imperial	Metric
1 fluid ounce	30 milliliters
2 fluid ounces	60 milliliters
3 fluid ounces	90 milliliters
4 fluid ounces	120 milliliters
5 fluid ounces	150 milliliters
6 fluid ounces	180 milliliters
7 fluid ounces	210 milliliters
8 fluid ounces	240 milliliters
44 fluid ounces	1¼ Liters
52 fluid ounces	1½ Liters
70 fluid ounces	2 Liters
88 fluid ounces	2½ Liters

10 fluid ounces	300 milliliters
12 fluid ounces	360 milliliters
14 fluid ounces	420 milliliters
16 fluid ounces	480 milliliters
18 fluid ounces	540 milliliters
20 fluid ounces	600 milliliters
24 fluid ounces	750 milliliters
35 fluid ounces	1 Liter

Sources References

https://nephcure.org/livingwithkidneydisease/diet-and-nutrition/renal-diet/#:~:text=A%20renal%20diet%20is%20one,to%20limit%20potassium%20and%20calcium.

https://share.upmc.com/2022/05/renal-diet/

https://www.davita.com/diet-nutrition/articles/advice/top-15-healthy-foods-for-people-with-kidney-disease

https://my.clevelandclinic.org/health/articles/15641-renal-diet-basics

https://www.niddk.nih.gov/health-information/kidney-disease/chronic-kidney-disease-ckd/eating-nutrition

https://www.niddk.nih.gov/health-information/kidney-disease/chronic-kidney-disease-ckd/eating-nutrition/nutrition-advanced-chronic-kidney-disease-adults

https://kidney.org.au/your-kidneys/living-with-kidney-disease/health-and-wellbeing/diet-nutrition

Conclusion

A renal diet is a diet that helps to protect the kidneys. Human kidneys are responsible for filtering waste from the blood, and a renal diet helps to reduce the amount of work they have to do. A renal diet is high in protein and low in salt, potassium, and phosphorus. It is important to follow a renal diet if you have kidney disease. This type of diet helps to slow down the progression of kidney disease and also improves your overall health.

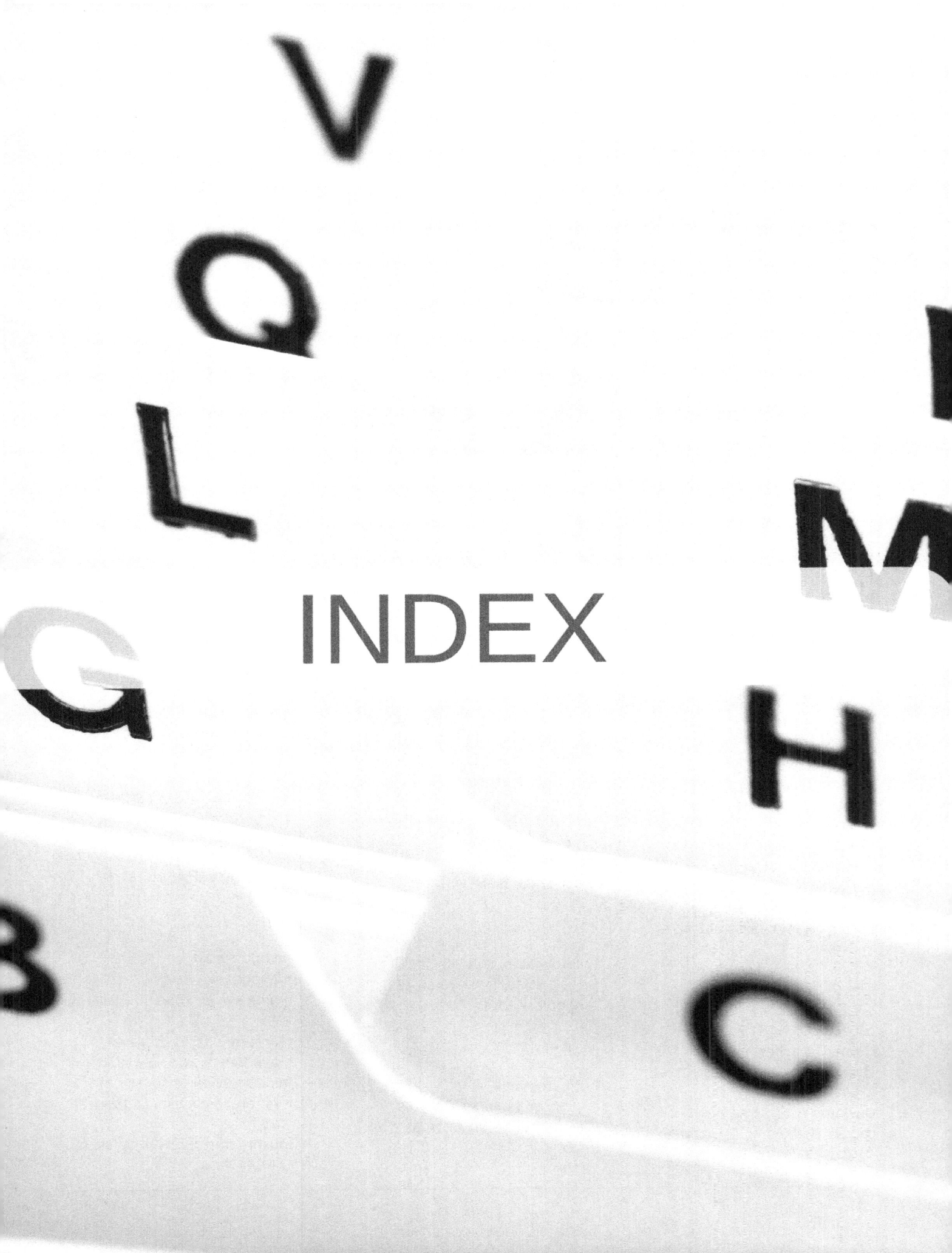

INDEX

Made in the USA
Coppell, TX
24 February 2023

13271438R20044